How to Succeed as a Leader

Edited by

Ruth Chambers
Kay Mohanna
Peter Spurgeon
and David Wall

Foreword by
David Nicholson

Radcliffe Publishing
Oxford • New York

Radcliffe Publishing Ltd
18 Marcham Road
Abingdon
Oxon OX14 1AA
United Kingdom

www.radcliffe-oxford.com
Electronic catalogue and worldwide online ordering facility.

British Library Cataloguing in Publication Data

A catalogue record for this book is available from the British Library.

ISBN-13: 978 1 84619 160 2

Typeset by Phoenix Photosetting, Chatham, Kent
Printed and bound by TJI Digital, Padstow, Cornwall

Contents

List of interactive exercises   v
Foreword   vii
Preface   ix
About the authors   xi

1 About leadership   1
   Peter Spurgeon

2 Communication skills as a leader   7
   Kay Mohanna

3 What are your learning needs?   15
   David Wall and Ruth Chambers

4 Tools and techniques to enable your personal effectiveness as a leader   25
   Ruth Chambers

5 Competencies of a good leader   33
   Robert Cragg and Peter Spurgeon

6 Leading the way as a good employer   41
   Ruth Chambers

7 Team leadership   47
   Hugh Flanagan and Veronica Wilkie

8 Change management   55
   Kay Mohanna

9 Finding time to be a leader   63
   Ruth Chambers

10 Organisational skills   69
    Kay Mohanna

11 Dealing with problems   77
    Veronica Wilkie and Hugh Flanagan

12 Being a leader through times of change   85
    Bev Norton

13 Leading research   91
    Ruth Chambers

14 Is it management or leadership?   97
    Peter Spurgeon and Robert Cragg

15 Leading amongst equals   101
    Peter Spurgeon and Robert Cragg

16 Growing new leaders   105
    Robert Cragg

Index   113

List of interactive exercises

Compare yourself with effective leaders   4
Mapping everyone's contributions   12
Self-assessment of your learning needs as a leader   22
Reflect on how effective you are from all angles   30
Gridlocked: analysing your competencies as a leader   37
Listening but not hearing   45
Team development and expectations   51
If at first you do not succeed ...   60
Time management is a lead issue   67
Analysing a stressful event   75
Get on the case when you are dealing with problems   82
All change – look to it   88
Undertake a significant event analysis of a problem relating to your
    research leadership   95
Getting the balance right   100
Finding an equally good way   104
Learning to cycle   110

Foreword

There has never been a more important time for the NHS to have strong leadership at all levels.

Over the past few years the NHS has been through an unparalleled period of change – driving through some of the most radical reforms since its inception.

The success – and the failures – we've experienced during that time can largely be tracked back to one thing: leadership. When I talk about leadership I don't just mean at Chief Executive level, but throughout NHS organisations, both at managerial and clinical levels.

This book provides a wealth of useful advice, tips and exercises that will help you challenge your own behaviour and the behaviour of those around you to improve and hone the skills needed to enhance your leadership qualities.

My own journey through the NHS began back in the early 1980s. After graduating from the National Management Training Scheme I worked in mental health services, mainly in Yorkshire, where I was involved in implementing the policy of closing the old asylums and developing services in the community. The lesson I learned from that period in my career was that it was possible to deliver big changes in the NHS if managers could harness the support of patients and their relatives.

The next phase of my career was in Doncaster, where I was appointed as the Chief Executive of Doncaster Royal Infirmary – one of the first wave NHS Trusts to break free from Whitehall control. The period I spent leading that organisation taught me the power of engaging clinicians to mobilise support for making change. I recognised that once clinicians and staff were engaged in change there was nothing stopping us from making real improvements to patient care.

And the third part of my career, which saw me as a Regional Director and Chief Executive in Trent and Birmingham, taught me the value of the system that underpins the NHS. Delivering change on a grand scale can only be achieved if all parts of the system are pointing in the right direction.

So my advice for any leader or aspiring leader in the NHS is to heed those three very important lessons that I learnt over more than 25 years in the NHS: engage with the public and patients so that everyone understands the direction of travel; work closely with clinicians so that everyone is pulling in the same direction; and ensure that you understand the implications that your decisions have on the system as a whole.

As an organisation with over 1.3 million staff the NHS has a huge amount of experience of leadership and this book draws on some of that experience from both managers and clinicians that will help provide you with both challenge and inspiration.

David Nicholson
NHS Chief Executive
October 2007

Preface

This is a book on leadership for any health professional or manager working in any setting where they have a leadership role and responsibilities. It should help you to understand what is expected from leaders – whether that is as a team leader in a practice or department, or as the chief executive of a large NHS trust or strategic health authority, or as a leader in education or research with an academic role. Leadership development will be relevant at all sorts of stages in your career, in various roles.

The book is all about presenting you with a practical approach to becoming a competent leader, to prepare you to lead in a positive way and realise your responsibilities as a leader.

The various chapters offer practical tools and approaches to enable you to work towards gaining the knowledge, skills and attributes, or competencies, of a good leader. You can identify and address the gaps in your knowledge and skills of which you were previously unaware – with a little help from others of course.

There is constant reorganisation and a changing culture in our health service. Good leadership is essential to address the changes required and take others with you so that the service can function effectively. There has been an amateurish approach to leadership in the NHS in the past, where people have become leaders without being prepared or trained for the role or supported in it.

Each chapter has been set out in the same way. Each starts with an introduction to the theme of the chapter and reinforces a key message with a telling quote. There follows a more in-depth section giving a succinct overview of the theme. The top tips share the live experiences of the experts. The subsequent answers to the frequently asked questions emphasise the way forward to effective leadership. The interactive exercise at the end of each chapter encourages the reader to put the wise words of the experts into practice in relation to their own circumstances. So, working through this book should give you a well founded grasp of what it takes to become a successful leader and guide you in applying what you read and learn.

Ruth Chambers
October 2007

About the authors

Ruth Chambers

Ruth has been a GP for more than 25 years and is currently the Director of Postgraduate GP Education at the Workforce Deanery, NHS West Midlands Strategic Health Authority. She has learnt a great deal about leadership from the various lead roles she has held at Stoke-on-Trent Teaching Primary Care Trust and as professor of primary care development at Staffordshire University, as well as in GP teams and in leading her many academic or development projects.

Robert Cragg

Robert currently works as a senior research associate at the Institute for Clinical Leadership, Warwick University. Since joining the NHS in 2001 as a graduate trainee, Robert has spent the last five years working in strategic and operational management roles across primary, secondary and tertiary care, as well as on secondment to the Commission for Health Improvement.

Currently Robert's role combines both training and research in the field of clinical leadership. He co-facilitates generic skills sessions for medics in training across the West Midlands, focusing on the acquisition of managerial and leadership competencies. His current research focus examines the role of clinical directors in the NHS and how organisational development strategies can be deployed to support such positions to enhance job satisfaction and managerial efficiency.

Hugh Flanagan

Hugh's career includes positions as a Board level executive director in the NHS, an academic researcher and postgraduate teacher on leadership, an NHS trust non-executive director and a Director of Consultancy for leadership and organisation development for a major national consultancy. He has worked across public and private sectors. His research includes an investigation into individual effectiveness in management and leadership in the public sector, with particular reference to the NHS. He has written generally on leadership and organisational development in health and public sector organisations and has undertaken postgraduate lecturing and senior management training in Sweden, Sri Lanka, Italy, France, Austria, Switzerland, Hong Kong and the Republic of Ireland.

Hugh is currently working on a range of leadership and management development programmes for doctors, and senior professionals and managers in the public sector. Other work includes programmes to develop partnership working, identifying and addressing causes of stress and poor performance in organisations, and new ways of assessing and developing leaders.

Kay Mohanna

Kay is principal lecturer in medical education at Staffordshire University where she is responsible for developing and delivering the Masters in Medical Education. She is also lead tutor on the 'Ethics for health care professionals' module. She is a GP partner in general practice, a GP trainer and vice chair of the Midland Faculty of the Royal College of General Practitioners. Most of what she knows about leadership has been learnt the hard way through making mistakes and trial and error. She has learnt a lot about effective leadership from the examples of others through her work in running a practice, teaching and training, the development of appraisal and careers support services.

Bev Norton

Bev has been a senior NHS manager for more than 25 years, with experience across the acute, community and primary care sectors of the health economy. Bev is currently a senior manager in Primary Care Development for NHS West Midlands Strategic Health Authority. The role involves leading on service development redesign, ensuring the delivery of national and local policy initiatives and effective development of primary care. Previously her roles have been to manage individuals and organisations through the changes of fund holding, transition of Primary Care Groups (PCGs) to Primary Care Trusts (PCTs), and Family Health Service Authorities (FHSAs) to Health Authorities, as well as the relocation of a hospital.

Peter Spurgeon

Peter is Director of the Institute for Clinical Leadership at the Medical School, University of Warwick. His current role involves research and provision of development activities relating to the role of doctors in management processes. The provision ranges from undergraduate level to the most senior clinicians in clinical and medical director roles.

For the past twenty years, Peter has worked at the Health Services Management Centre, University of Birmingham; where as well as being Centre Director he had a number of lead roles such as Head of Research and Consultancy. He is an experienced health services researcher with a particular interest in personal and organisational development.

David Wall

David is deputy regional postgraduate dean in the Workforce Deanery, NHS West Midlands, and professor of medical education at Staffordshire University. He has been a general practitioner in Sutton Coldfield for 30 years, since starting there in 1974. He has a Masters degree in Medical Education from the University of Dundee. He has just obtained a PhD in Education from the University of Birmingham. His main work in the Workforce Deanery is with doctors and dentists in difficulty, educational research and faculty development.

Veronica Wilkie

Veronica is a GP in Droitwich, Worcestershire. She is a GP trainer and has been a clinical tutor with the NHS West Midlands Workforce Deanery for 10 years. She currently develops courses and researches on leadership, management and evidence based practice for doctors and dentists in training as a clinical fellow with the Institute for Clinical Leadership at the University of Warwick.

Chapter 1

About leadership

Peter Spurgeon

Introduction

The NHS has experienced a prolonged period of upheaval; most notably in the form of seemingly constant structural change. The current focus upon new ways of delivering services associated with stringent financial controls and unprecedented job losses with yet further organisational restructuring is as great as any change experienced by the NHS to date. Previous failures or problems in the NHS are often blamed on a lack of leadership, whilst the demand for good leadership is said to be at a premium as the only way to cope with the present challenges.

The term *leadership* when used in this very general way can come to mean almost whatever you want it to mean, and is on the whole unhelpful to those who aspire to contribute through their own leadership capacity in a variety of roles. Here, we offer you some insight and understanding as to how leadership operates in a variety of contexts.

> Ros Taylor, a business psychologist and author, emphasises the importance of the extent of infrastructure support for leaders so that they can be effective:
>
> I have found the standards of leadership in the NHS extremely high. Leadership is about being comfortable putting yourself out in front, wanting to make a difference and having some answers about how to do that. It is not about organising your own diary or typing up memos. There are some fantastic thinkers in the NHS who end up doing mundane tasks because they don't have a PA. The amount of stress this causes is immense.[1]

Leadership: what do we know?

The literature on leadership is vast, running to millions of citations. Inevitably in such a prolific field the definitions used are variable. Clarity about just what is meant by the term *leadership* is lacking. There is a tendency to confuse the question: *Who are leaders?* with *What do leaders do?* The former approach leads to an unending series of lists of personal qualities that an individual, designated as a leader might possess. Sadly as you line yourself up against the list you will fall short. The paragon matching up to all the virtues described does not exist. If they did, they would be unlikely to be applying for a job where such lists are often to be found.

The reality is that you may possess some of these personal characteristics to some degree – but just how much of each do you need to be a leader? Since individuals do emerge as leaders with an almost infinite set of combinations of personal characteristics then your first conclusion must be that there are lots of ways in which people can lead and that no single universal set of characteristics is required. This is helpful in two ways:

1 as individuals we can all make a contribution as leaders in different ways
2 when reading the many descriptions of leadership it is entirely legitimate to choose a model that fits with your own personal make-up or chosen model of leadership. No proposed model is right. But elements can be adapted and grafted onto others to offer you an approach to being a leader that is comfortable and compatible with your own individual resources.

The fascination with leadership in a personal capacity is in part a recognition of the interpersonal nature of leadership, i.e. how we as leaders have an impact on others. It also reflects a key distinction between management and leadership. Management requires a degree of rationality and is aimed at efficiency. Leadership by its nature is more affective in that it is about generating followership, by inspiring, motivating, energising or convincing others that the direction or goal identified is worthwhile and appropriately demanding of their commitment.

The glaring weakness of the personal characteristics approach, even beyond clarifying which characteristics are needed, is that it does not really offer any insight to the aspiring leader as to what leadership involves in terms of activities or behaviours. Therefore the second overall question to emerge around leadership is, *What do leaders actually do?* This behavioural approach typically leads to a set of leadership competencies or behaviours which taken together represent the repertoire of actions an individual can take. The Leadership Qualities Framework (LQF) recently developed specifically for the NHS is an example of this approach.[2] The LQF and competencies are discussed as a specific aspect of leadership in Chapter 5.

Although the number of competency frameworks is growing with the risk of creating confusion about their relative merits, the competency approach has two particular advantages:

● although the language of competency frameworks often looks different there is frequently a great deal of underlying overlap in what competencies are being described
● even when particular competencies seem to be demanding, they are accessible to the individual and offer the prospect of being acquired through appropriate training and development opportunities.

A third way that some people think about leadership is to define it in terms of outcome such that if a unit or group is successful then they must by definition have experienced good leadership and vice versa. An example of this is the published study conducted by the Hay Group.[3,4] The overall conclusion of the study was that effective ward management led to fewer drug errors, higher patient satisfaction and lower staff absenteeism and turnover. Whilst the differences reported in some of these areas was substantial it is worth noting that 'effective and poor-performing managers were identified by analysing results in three areas for the 12 months before the study. These were: the number and severity of drug errors, the frequency and nature of patient complaints, staff turnover and absenteeism.' Thus the product or outcome is itself used to define leadership. The study also reported that the more effective leaders used a greater variety of styles of leadership ranging from coercive, to democratic to coaching styles.[5] The real point is that effectiveness is associated with being able to link a leadership approach to the nature of the problem and people involved.

We see many examples of leaders being defined by outcome in various sectors and also the fallacy of the approach. Successful companies by definition must be effectively led but when leaders are recruited to a new setting they often fail. The lessons about leadership would seem to be that:

- it is fundamentally about influencing others
- each individual can make a contribution as a leader in an enormous variety of ways based on their personal attributes and the style adopted
- the setting, context and nature of the people being influenced make a great difference to what is classed as effective leadership.[5]

Top tips

- Be aware of the context in which you exercise leadership – its history and values.
- Understand the task so that it is apparent what type of leadership might be needed and should work best.
- Develop your own self-awareness so that you can build on your strengths, and develop a style that suits you.
- The best leaders can adapt their leadership style to the needs of the situation.
- Leadership can be offered at all sorts of levels in the organisation and there is a need to create room for both individuals and the organisation to flourish.
- Leading is a complex matter, so recognise the contributions made by those around you.
- Recognise and encourage talent. To do so should not be a threat but will make you a better leader.
- Be clear about your focus and what you are trying to achieve as a leader.
- Be willing to communicate to others what is happening and how you are going to do it over and over again.
- Get feedback from others as to the leadership style that you commonly use – how well it seems to work in your everyday work and leadership roles. This might be informal feedback or structured from a multisource feedback exercise (*see* Chapter 3).
- Become familiar with the various approaches to leadership – read all about them and reflect on what suits you and your circumstances.[2,3,4,5]
- Try to protect time for your development as a leader. Be strict with yourself about prioritising your learning in the midst of all your other commitments and pressures. Negotiate with your employers or colleagues for time out, and funding for pursuing training activities.

Frequently asked questions and answers

Q. *I have recently joined a new practice as a GP partner. Overall the practice has survived rather than been successful. I sense people looking at me to lead improvements but I am not really clear how to go about it. What approach should I take?*

A. This is a context whereby someone is expected to provide leadership because of their seniority and expertise but where they have probably had little or no training in the skills of leadership. It is partly an issue of confidence, i.e. feeling that it is reasonable for you to start suggesting what should change and how staff should go about things. It is also an error to believe that there exists some prescriptive guide to leadership that will tell you what to do. The most likely way to be effective as a leader in this setting is to believe in yourself in establishing a lead in a way that feels comfortable and most like your own preferred style. But be aware of the reaction of others and be sensitive enough to adapt your approach if it is triggering difficulties.

Q. *How do I decide if I have leadership qualities?*

A. The key is a combination of self-awareness and self-insight – know what you are like, what your strengths and weaknesses are – and then link this to some kind of feedback. The feedback can be derived from many sources – from trusted colleagues who can tell you how you are seen by others; from a psychometric profile carried out by someone competent to give you sensitive feedback and guidance as to how you might develop certain skills; or by attending a formal course that offers you insight into the models of leadership that exist and allows you and other participants to practise some leadership behaviours. Then you can reflect how this works out in real life when you try them out back in your workplace.

Interactive exercise: compare yourself with effective leaders

Ideally this exercise should be carried out with two or three colleagues. You should list:

1 three examples of leadership behaviour that you have experienced that you believe made a difference to the outcome in a particular situation. Make sure the list is of behaviours, not personal characteristics
2 identify three people who you believe have leadership capacity. Describe what it is about them that defines them as leaders.

Compare the types of information obtained from the two tasks and then consider whether you behave in ways like those described in (1) or possess characteristics such as those described in (2). If not, think about how you could exercise leadership from a different basis from these two approaches.

It would then be good to discuss your reflections with a colleague or mentor and get their perspectives before making a plan to try out these leadership styles. You could meet up and discuss how your leadership worked out later on.

References

1   Taylor R. Personal communication; 2006.
2   NHS Leadership Centre. *Leadership Qualities Framework*; 2002. www.nhsleadership qualities.nhs.uk.

3   Carlisle D. Outside Edge. *Health Serv J.* 2006; **116**(6010): 34–6.
4   Hay Group. *In tune with the team;* 2006 www.haygroup.com.
5   Rushmer R, Kelly D, Lough M, *et al.* Introducing the Learning Practice III Leadership: empowerment, protected time and reflective practice as core contextual conditions. *J Eval Clin Pract.* 2004; **10**(3): 399–405.

Chapter 2

Communication skills as a leader

Kay Mohanna

Introduction

Managing and leading teams requires many skills that are similar to those used in the clinical setting. Communication skills are chief amongst these. Leaders need to be comfortable working with, and talking to, staff or colleagues individually or collectively, with executive decision makers – in the NHS as a whole as well as to individual patients. You might think that you are a good communicator and be baffled when others do not understand what is perfectly clear to you. It is sometimes said that a message is the reaction it evokes in the listener – but we tend to think of it as being what we say. In the gap between leader and team, funny things can happen to that message if you are not careful.

This chapter covers some of the key communication skills required to be a good leader:

- creating rapport
- challenging
- managing conflict
- influencing – including disseminating information/reasons for action
- negotiating – including discussing strategies to gain ownership
- understanding that language is more than just words.

> There is nothing more demoralising than a leader who cannot clearly articulate why we are doing what we are doing.
>
> Kouzes and Poisner[1]

What makes effective communication by a leader?

Good leadership is easier to recognise than define, but there are certain characteristic, observable attributes and some of these are demonstrated in the quality of communication between leaders and their team members. Good leaders are followed chiefly because people trust and respect them. This arises out of qualities such as integrity, honesty, humility, courage, commitment, sincerity, passion, confidence, positivity, wisdom, determination, compassion and sensitivity. In this respect, leadership can be distinguished from management – although the distinction may be false and both activities have large areas of overlap. But management relies more on planning, organisational and team development and perhaps less on personal integrity and quality of communication.

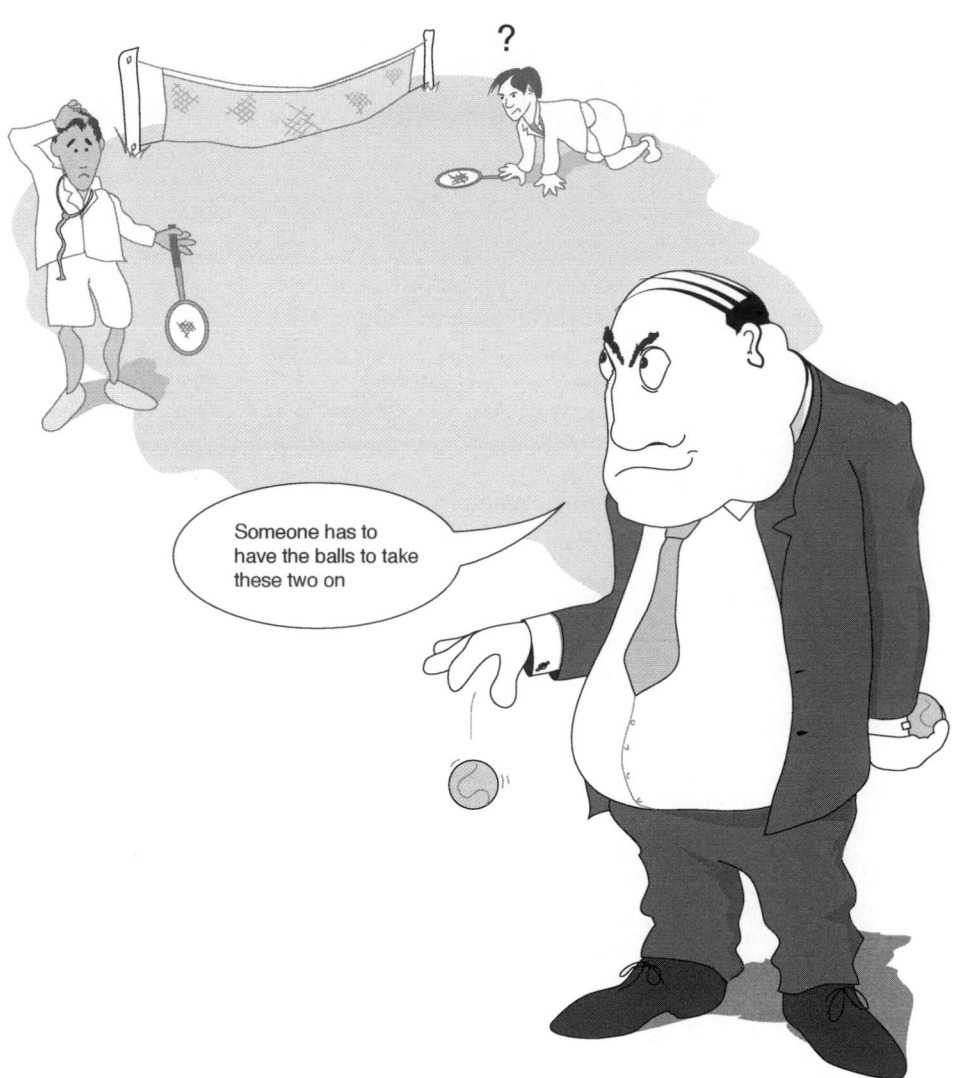

Good leaders:

- listen
- consult
- involve
- explain *why*, as well as *what*, needs to be done.

Leadership requires you to develop a *rapport* with team members. You can do this by creating a conducive environment, where ideas are welcomed and contributions are valued. But additionally you need to think about the language that you use. The use of jargon and ill-defined terms can lead to confusion and risk isolating or excluding team members. It can be helpful, as appropriate, to actively alter the balance of your language from the dogmatic to provisional and from judgemental to descriptive. Statements such as 'You will do this action by that date', become 'Let's aim to try out this plan and look at it again by this date'. Comments on suggestions change from 'That's a rubbish idea' to 'I think you might see this (specific) unwanted outcome if you try that'.

Effective leaders try to minimise comments about individuals and stick to issues. They recognise and interpret their own feelings without necessarily describing them to others. All these skills allow them to develop a healthy rapport with colleagues and build well functioning teams.

Good leaders challenge. They challenge others and motivate them to reach higher levels of personal and organisational achievement and they challenge poor performance when they see it. This is related to the skill of managing conflict. In these situations, there might be a failure to implement a change due to poor planning, or team disputes; individual team members might be actively trying to derail the process or acting incompetently and putting the project at risk. It is important to tackle areas of conflict when they arise, difficult though it often is, because left unchecked resentment and general discomfort can build up, leading to factions developing and the taking of sides. It can help to consider these questions:

- why has this happened at this stage?
- what aspects of the personnel, the issues and the timing are adding to the conflict? (These need to be identified and reduced).
- what factors are helping to minimise the conflict? (These need to be developed).
- can you get back on track, or is this project doomed?

Good leaders act decisively to make decisions about situations of conflict, give clear orders about actions to remediate conflict situations, or abandon plans and have a rethink.

Influencing and negotiating are related skills. Negotiation can be described as 'influencing with integrity'.

Negotiating may be defined as formal discussion between people who are trying to reach an agreement. Good leaders recognise that the party they are negotiating with is their opposite, rather than their opponent. If you ride roughshod over your opposite number, you may win this time, but you risk using up any goodwill and incurring problems next time. Negotiations should continue to develop good relationships not destroy them. Consider your opposite's proposal as just another option. Never insult, irritate, blame or make accusations.

Take care about how you bring up your idea; try stating the background reasons and then the proposal, rather than the other way round. Emphasise existing areas of agreement and try to see things from your opposite's perspective. In an impasse, maintain your objectives, not your position and identify points of agreement. It may be important to identify intentions and negative consequences of certain paths of action. Good negotiators will maintain a degree of flexibility. Identifying your bottom line and the gap between this and your preferred outcome represents your 'settlement range' for the negotiations.

In preparation for a negotiation it pays to:

- be clear about your objectives – stick to your bottom line
- know your opposite's objectives
- know your opposite's hierarchy of values
- know about the external factors influencing negotiation – such as the implications regarding resources
- have a list of acceptable options
- take care over arrangements in relation to organising an appropriate venue and the timing.

Interpreting others' meanings

Effective communication is facilitated by paying attention to personal integrity, and having a behavioural understanding of what good communication is like.

A lot of communication between leaders and team members is implicit, just as between everyone else in their daily interactions. You assume a degree of mutual understanding based on norms, experiences and 'the way things are'. The risk in this is that there are times when you come into contact with people and situations where you don't all have the same understanding of how things are (or how they should be). This 'cultural familiarity' is lost – an understanding of how your business or organisation works, what behaviours are expected and what rewarded. So often in meetings much is taken for granted; not just the specialist language that is used, but what is left unsaid and the 'rules' governing interactions, so that the sense of the discussion goes over some people's heads.

This thinking can be extended to consider your internal 'map' that represents your personal model of how you perceive the world itself to be. This map develops in response to your personal experiences and observations. And the key thing is that these maps are different for all of us. You don't operate directly on the world but through your maps and models. Failing to recognise this difference can lead to dysfunctional communication.

The effect of this 'model making' can be heard in your speech and good leaders can detect this. So avoid falling into the trap of making assumptions about shared understanding. In the same way that your model making turns your experience into your understanding of reality, the spoken word represents an inner, deeper meaning. Differences in your understanding show themselves in three main ways in your speech which, in neurolinguistic programming (NLP),[2] are called deletions, generalisations and distortions. You can analyse your communication with an eye to the impact of these three effects.

A deletion may be of a simple word or words, e.g. 'I am confused' (about what?), of nouns or verbs, e.g. 'They always get in my way' (who gets in your way?) of unspecified relations 'She is the best one for the job' (better than whom?) or of unspecified processes, e.g. 'I don't like people being unclear' (unclear to whom, about what?).

Linguistic generalisations take isolated examples and let them represent an entire category. This can be positive as it enables you to make rules to live by, but you need to check the basis on which they are made. 'Nobody listens to my ideas.' (What, no one person has ever listened to you?) 'I have to consider the feelings of others.' (What will happen if you don't?) 'It's wrong to slow the group down.' (Who says? Wrong in what way? For whom?)

Linguistic distortions represent a shift that has been made in how you represent sensory data. One good outcome of this is to allow you to imagine a wide range of possibilities. When it becomes a problem is when you assume that one observation is inextricably linked to a given meaning, e.g. 'Poor eye contact means you are a shifty person.' (But doesn't it mean that you are respectful of your elders in some countries?)

You can learn to recognise the deletions, distortions and generalisations that occur in speech to clarify meaning and understanding.

Top tips

Good leaders communicate well by:

- listening, i.e. hearing, valuing and showing that they have heard what is said to them
- recognising and responding to emotion in themselves and others
- avoiding building barriers by excessive use of jargon
- understanding when formal or informal forms of communication are appropriate
- creating opportunities where all team members feel able to contribute
- appreciating the diversity of experience, opinion and knowledge of all team members
- using shared decision making to promote joint ownership of outcomes
- avoiding game-playing, and recognising it when it occurs in others
- confronting conflict and acting decisively to trouble-shoot and problem-solve
- developing communication networks, e.g. email groups, newsletters, staff meetings
- sharing news and notifying others promptly about changes
- being readily available to and contactable by others.

Frequently asked questions and answers

Q. *Why is my team so hopeless at carrying out instructions? There is always such resistance to new ideas that I feel as though I am hitting my head against a brick wall at times.*
A. What has been your team's previous experience of change? This could be an anxiety provoking time for them. Could you be a bit less authoritarian and a bit more collaborative? Cooperation within teams can break down as a result of inconsistent management, lack of guidance, poor communication or lack of support – real or perceived. A good team leader will encourage rather than impose change and ensure that teams feel consulted, involved, and can see the reason for change.

Q. *How come when I try to involve team members in developing ideas I am met with a wall of silence? How can I get more involvement?*
A. It can be challenging to have to come up with ideas when you don't know how they will be received. Maybe you will be laughed at, or worse, ignored. Try to develop a culture that is frank and supportive where people can speak out and their ideas be valued. This means encouraging quieter members by arranging small working groups within the team and laying out some ground rules about how suggestions will be received by all team members. Power issues can get in the way too. Do you have different team members with varying seniority? This can affect how willing people are to speak out.

Interactive exercise: mapping everyone's contributions

Try this communication exercise next time you are in a meeting that you are not chairing and where you have a chance to watch the process rather than concentrate on the content. It works best in small- to medium-sized meetings of four to six people.

1 Sketch out a map of where people are sitting around the table.
2 As they talk, connect the participants with lines that represent the flow of contributions to the debate.
3 Label each line with the two types of communication that might occur:
   – contributions that affect the group dynamics, that keep the group on task or are destructive to the group
   – those that address the topic.
   Some members will talk more than others and they will have several lines coming from them.
4 Other observations you might make include:
   – thinking aloud
   – clarifying the task
   – sharing ideas
   – testing theories
   – challenging others
   – offering solutions.

Some members will nurture others and bring them into the discussion: 'What do you think John? This is your area of expertise.' Some members will seek to clarify meaning – echoing, paraphrasing, reflecting. Some will summarise what has been said. Some will draw attention to constraints: 'Come on we have got to get this sorted by 11a.m.' or 'That will cost too much.'

Note your own contribution too (if it is not too affected by the exercise!). Are you a content or a process person in group discussions?

Which type of contributions helped the group to solve the task? What got in the way? Has a natural leader emerged?

When you have got the hang of keeping track of communication in a meeting, you could try doing it when you are leading a discussion. That way you may gain insights into your personal style of leadership. Be careful to avoid laying yourself open to the charge that you are not keeping up with the content of the meeting though!

Acknowledgment

Our understanding of the 'meta model '– the application of the presuppositions of NLP to communication – was considerably advanced by conversations with, and the work of, Dr Jonas Millar.

References

1   Kouzes J, Poisner B. *The Leadership Challenge*. 3rd ed. San Francisco: Jossey Bass; 2002.
2   Walker L. *Consulting with NLP*. Oxford: Radcliffe Medical Press; 2002.

Chapter 3

What are your learning needs?

David Wall and Ruth Chambers

Introduction

Leadership skills' training is an important area for many health professionals and managers working for the NHS. General practitioners, dentists, pharmacists and other independent contractors are self-employed professionals running their own businesses, and so must take business decisions on behalf of themselves, their staff and their patients. Leadership skills training has become even more important for GPs, dentists and pharmacists since the advent of their latest NHS contracts, when dealing with the many changes that have been heaped upon them as part and parcel of working in the NHS. If we in the health professions needed good leadership before, then we certainly do now.

> The fundamental problem in our NHS is lack of true medical leadership. Be it about patients' safety, medical errors, clinical governance, career progression, the MMC (Modernising Medical Careers) initiative or performance management of doctors. Creating institutions like NPSA (the National Patient Safety Agency) and so on are good ideas provided these ideas are translated into reality at the coalface. That is the problem. Unless the NHS appoints the right people to do the right job and gives them the right tools, resources and training and then performance manages them, things are not going to change.
>
> (Senior doctor's frustrated rant in an electronic discussion forum)

Finding out what you might want to learn about to become a better leader

A formal learning needs analysis may involve a third party undertaking interviews with, or seeking feedback from colleagues, surveys of all those affected by your role, and performance data relating directly to you as an individual or concerning others for whom you are responsible in a lead role. You could fix on what core competencies of a leader you are aiming for by describing the knowledge, skills, attributes or behaviour you need to be an effective leader – in order to analyse your developmental needs.

Range of methods to identify your learning needs

You may decide to use a few selected methods to identify your learning needs in respect of leadership. One approach is triangulation. If you have three pieces of evidence pointing in a particular direction then it is probably true. For this type of combined assessment, you might use for example:

- a self-assessment using a rating scale to assess your skills and attitudes, or peer review
- a strengths, weaknesses, opportunities and threats (SWOT) analysis
- some type of feedback on your performance and attitude relating to your leadership: e.g. significant event audit; constructive feedback with peer observation; 360° or multisource feedback from colleagues of all seniority and users of your service; review of team difficulties with colleagues to recognise where a lack of competence (you as a leader or them as team members), accessibility, inadequate communication or use of resources has affected the process or outcome for those affected
- areas where you are challenged in a leadership role to justify why you do what you do – by self-reflection or in discussion with another person, e.g. a colleague or mentor
- audit of protocols and guidelines for checking how well procedures are followed; reviews of how well resources, access and availability are managed.

Group and summarise your learning needs from the exercises you have carried out. Grade them according to how you weight them. You may put one at a higher priority because it fits in with learning needs established from another section, or put another lower because it does not fit in with other activities that you will put into your learning plan for the next twelve months. Record what learning needs assessments have contributed to establishing your leadership needs, and which ones you have decided to concentrate on now.

Self-assessment

Ramsden has described seven key leadership attributes.[1] You can self-assess your own strengths and preferences using the questionnaire developed from these descriptors (*see* the interactive exercise on page 22). These are *fair and efficient management, development and recognition, interpersonal skills, strategy and vision, transformation and collaborative leadership, leadership for teaching* and *leadership for research*. For each of these seven items, there are descriptors to explain and amplify each of the attributes. These are:

1 **fair and efficient management**: this means delegating fairly, managing resources effectively, collaborating with others, maintaining fairness and openness in decision making, being well organised, tackling problems quickly and effectively, and getting things done
2 **development and recognition**: this is readily acknowledging the contributions of others, working to develop others as leaders, helping people to develop their full potential, providing opportunities to help others
3 **interpersonal skills**: this is about developing a good communication style, being open and approachable, giving feedback constructively, being welcoming to others, being clear with expectations and honesty
4 **strategy and vision**: this involves building a good reputation for the organisation, seeing the big picture, creating a shared vision, bringing in new resources, understanding different viewpoints and encouraging new thinking

5 **transformational and collaborative leadership**: this includes motivating people, encouraging participation, welcoming questions, setting challenges, encouraging the sharing of ideas and learning positively from mistakes

6 **leadership for teaching**: this encompasses conveying an excitement for teaching, inspiring respect as a teacher, bringing in new ideas for teaching, and being keen to improve teaching

7 **leadership for research**: this involves relaying an excitement for research, inspiring respect as a researcher, helping colleagues develop as researchers, and creating a supportive climate for research.

It is uncommon for healthcare professionals to prioritise learning needs relating to leadership over other aspects of their work. The following quote from a PCT appraisal lead illustrates this; only one of the 30 GPs who had been appraised in the previous year had recognised a need for them to learn more about leadership, despite all being leaders in some aspects of their everyday role – neither had their appraisers realised this at the appraisal interview.

> Looking for leadership training needs in 30 appraisal forms (Form 4 returns) produced remarkably little … There was not a distinction between management and leadership which I think are quite different things. So no one declared themselves as aspiring to lead, let alone identifying what training they would need. Some form of learning needs in relation to management/leadership skills was raised by three of the 30 GPs only; two related to appraisal processes for their staff and the other was a rather ill defined 'practice organisation' … Appraisals haven't brought out any request for leadership courses or been noted in personal development plans (PDPs).

Learning from mistakes

One way of determining your and others' learning needs is about learning from mistakes – as an organisation, or you as an individual. For that to happen, it is vital that errors or 'near misses' can be reported without fear of recrimination. And for such a culture to be prevalent, requires good leadership. It can be a difficult balance to achieve, encouraging people to report such errors or near misses, but not tolerating poor performance. The culture at work should be open and leaders should encourage everyone to feel responsible for maintaining high standards. Learning from errors and near misses requires insight and learning, and once that has been gained, evidence of changed behaviour and practice – within the organisation and throughout the workforce. Where insight into causes and effects of adverse incidents is not present it is essential to have robust risk management and critical incident analysis systems in place. The key to success in this area is good leadership to ensure that the learning from such systems is fed directly into the corporate planning process and your own and others' personal development plans.

Significant event audit (SEA)

Significant event auditing is a structured approach to reviewing events that have occurred and provides a rich source of material for identifying your learning needs as a leader as well as improving services. SEA uses teamworking to high-light any problems with the relationships between colleagues and staff and to provide agreed solutions that can be implemented. But it requires good leader-ship to trigger the SEA and conduct the SEA cycle in such a way that others feel comfortable and confident in joining in.

To carry out a SEA, a group of people involved in that event should meet together. They should agree a review of the event, adopting a no-blame attitude and mutual trust and respect for each other. Confidentiality rules must be set out right from the start. All must agree on confidentiality about what is discussed and any reporting must be anonymised. The members of the group discuss the events and some or all of the following:

- management of the event
- any opportunities for prevention
- learning needs and how these will be addressed
- follow up
- implications for those involved, e.g. if a patient is concerned, their relatives and the community
- actions of the clinical and non-clinical members of the team
- what actions should be taken as a result of the review
- how the actions (if required) will be evaluated or monitored.

Some significant events are adverse incidents. These are events where something has clearly gone wrong, and there is a need to establish what happened, what was preventable and what changes are needed. Some adverse incidents reveal only minor risks or ones that would occur extremely infrequently and will be judged by the team as not requiring any changes. By contrast an adverse event that is very serious, however rare, may require action. In hospital settings, a range of confidential reviews such as those relating to maternity events, deaths and sui-cides provide useful occasions to review your role as a leader and of the quality of teamworking and other issues.

360° or multisource feedback[2]

This type of exercise collects together perceptions from a number of different par-ticipants as in Box 3.1. They should encompass a range of people with whom you work within and outside your organisation and team, and those who come into contact with you in your leadership role.

The wider the spread of people giving feedback, the more rounded the picture. There will be a minimum number of respondents required for the results of the feedback exercise to be considered valid; for instance maybe ten or fifteen. An independent person then collects and collates the questionnaires and discusses the results with the individual. The main disadvantage of this method is that it can sometimes be spoilt by malicious comments against which individuals cannot readily defend themselves. So the quality and presentation of the feedback is key. There are many tools available and being developed.

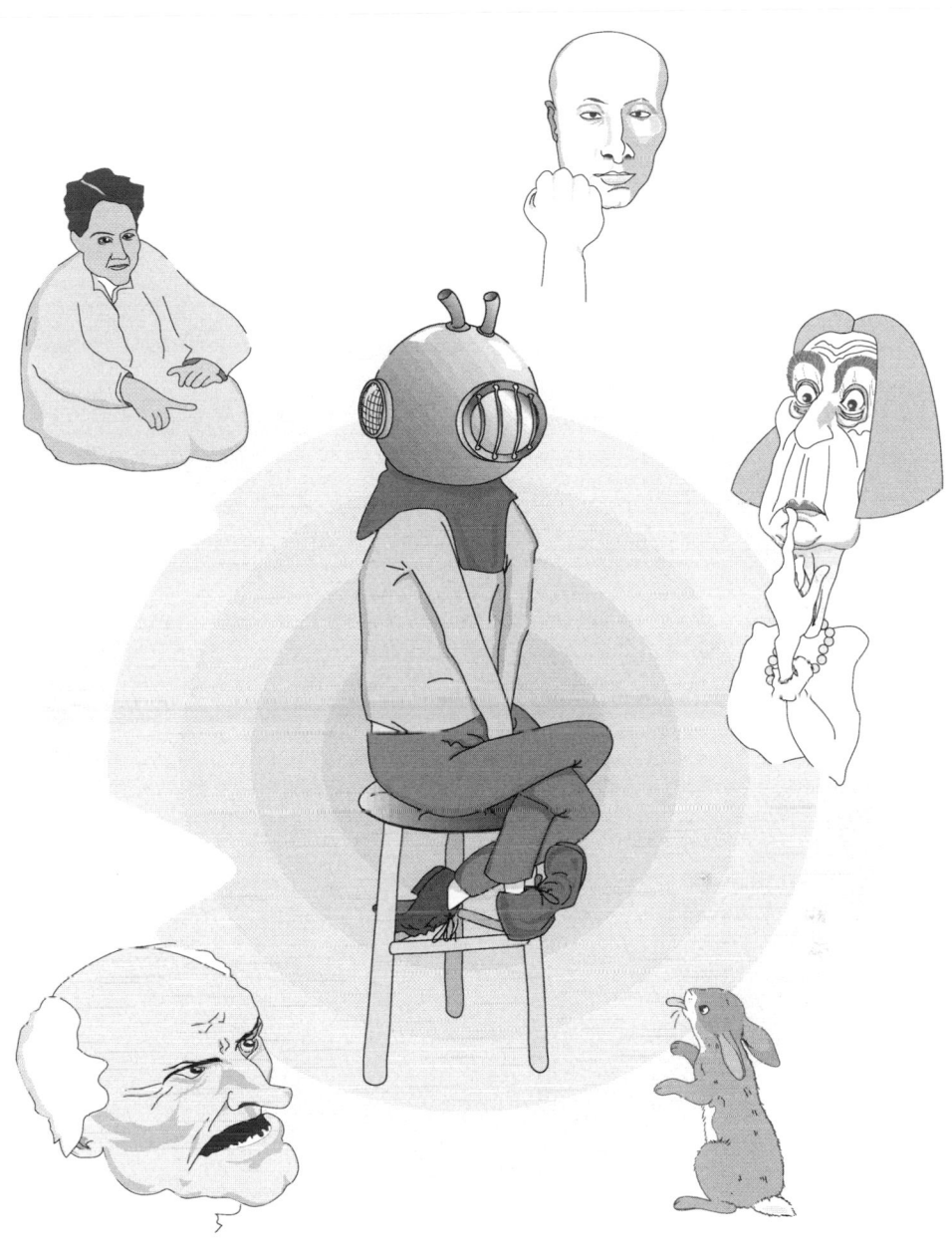

Hearing what others think of you can be upsetting, if not handled well.

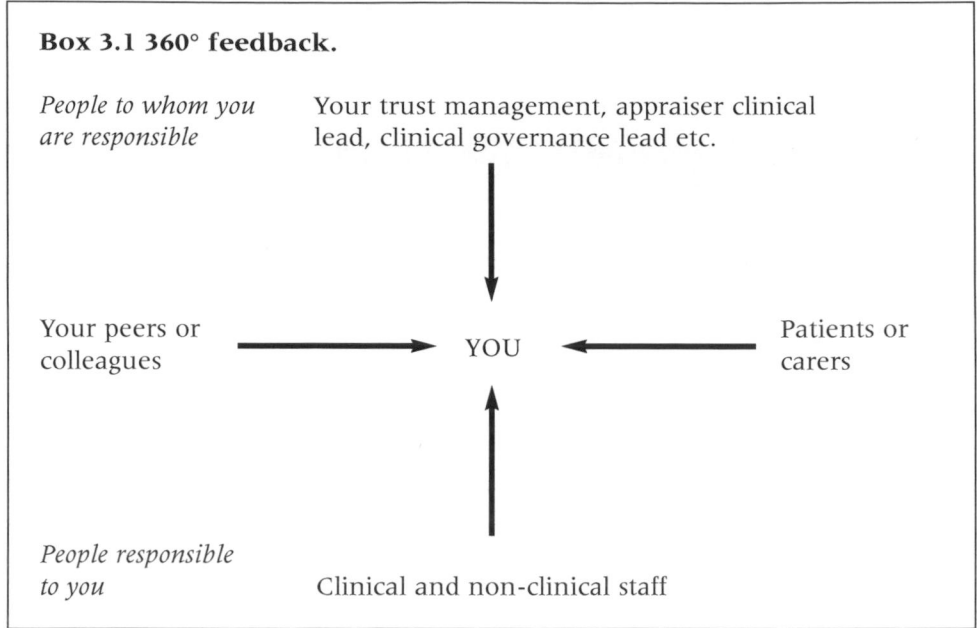

Box 3.1 360° feedback.

*People to whom you
are responsible*   Your trust management, appraiser clinical
                    lead, clinical governance lead etc.

Your peers or   YOU   Patients or
colleagues   carers

*People responsible
to you*   Clinical and non-clinical staff

Top tips

1 When analysing your learning needs in relation to leadership:
   - keep in mind that the health service exists to provide care for patients. So your learning needs relate to the nature of a leadership role that prioritises the needs of patients
   - gather information about what your organisation or the NHS in general requires from you in your leadership role – their priorities and your place in the organisational structure; balance that wider view with your personal perspectives
   - plan for the future; the development of your current role and services you anticipate being provided
   - if you have identified a learning need by several different methods of assessment then it will have a higher priority than something you have only identified once
   - read through the relevant chapters of this book first (note: actually they are all relevant – read the whole book through!) before describing the type of leader you are/want to be and the quality/nature of service you expect to deliver with the team(s) involved
   - make sure that you get objective feedback from others in any learning needs analysis – from an organisational angle and in relation to your personal performance and behaviour.
2 When planning how you will address your learning needs think about:
   - is your aim clear?
   - are you able to define your objectives?
   - can you justify spending time and effort on that topic? Is it serious enough or occurring sufficiently often to warrant the time spent?

- are the time and resources for learning about that topic available – in your preferred format (e.g. an action learning set) or will other 'cheaper' learning formats fulfil your needs (e.g. reading a handbook without peer discussion and challenge)?
- will learning about that topic make a difference to the leadership you can provide for your team?
- how does this topic fit in with other topics you have identified that you should learn more about, not necessarily to do with leadership but concerning other components of your work?

Frequently asked questions and answers

Q. *I'm a busy person. I have got patients queuing up to see me and am drowning in paperwork; my staff continually interrupt me with urgent problems that only I can solve. How can I justify doing a time consuming learning needs analysis of my leadership role when I have got lots more pressing things to do?*
A. It does sound like you need to step back and review what you are doing and how you organise your working life – to check that you are working effectively. So any time spent on analysing your learning needs should be recouped many times over by introducing better ways of working. If you can act as an effective leader your team may become more autonomous and interrupt you less often to demand that you solve their problems, for instance.

Look at the NHS Leadership Qualities Framework (www.nhsleadershipqualities. nhs.uk) and imagine how good you will feel when you have enhanced your self belief, self awareness, self management and drive for improvement, whilst maintaining your personal integrity. Maybe your organisation could register you on a national leadership development programme so that you have protected time for development (such as the British Association of Medical Managers' Fit to Lead programme www.fittolead.co.uk)? You could find a colleague in a similar leadership position to act as a buddy and both work together to analyse your learning needs – that should help you to agree and keep to a timetable, give you an independent view of your needs, allow you to share the gathering of information about corporate priorities and plans. Start with the self-assessment exercise on page 22 and compare yourself with others' self-evaluations in Table 3.1 to kick-start your learning needs analysis. Once you get into it, you will see that the potential benefits outweigh your effort.

Q. *How can I distinguish between the sort of competencies that I need in starting out in my new role as a leader in my team, compared to those that an established leader in our trust would need to have?*
A. Your picture of yourself as a competent leader will probably reflect a number of common themes:

- knowledge, understanding and judgement
- a range of skills – cognitive, technical or psychomotor and inter-personal
- a range of personal attributes.

These will be similar for a leader of any seniority or working in a range of settings. The established leader will have a much more complex role across an organisation, dealing with other stakeholders and with more external pressures than you are likely to have in your team with a more limited scope and set of responsibilities. You will aim to be competent as a leader of your team, handling the usual requirements placed on you and the team. As you learn more and take on more senior leadership roles you will need to learn to cope with the unexpected. Then perform well as a leader when in extreme conflict situations or there is a clash of values with what is being required of you. Some describe this transition as the 'novice to expert' pathway, starting from where you are now being aware of the knowledge, skills and attitudes you need as a team leader, to gaining those competencies and performing well under normal conditions, to becoming more proficient then expert as you cope with a wider set of responsibilities and unpredictable events or demands.[3]

Interactive exercise: self-assessment of your learning needs as a leader

Step 1: self-assessment – look back at the seven attributes of a leader according to Ramsden[1] and reflect how your own style matches up.

Step 2: write down a few reflective statements about this using a simple reflective template, as in Table 3.1.

Table 3.1 Self-reflection on your learning needs in respect of your leadership style.

Date *Place*	*Questions raised by what has gone on*
Direct observations and recalled events written as recollections as soon as possible – to include descriptions and personal responses both felt and intellectual	
	Implications for next action/future Implications for practice/intentions
	Additional later reflections

References

1 Ramsden P. *Learning to Lead in Higher Education*. London: Routledge; 1998.
2 King J. Career focus: 360° appraisal. *BMJ*. 2002; **324**: S195.
3 Benner P. *Novice to Expert*. London: Addison Welsley; 1984.

Chapter 4

Tools and techniques to enable your personal effectiveness as a leader

Ruth Chambers

Introduction

The techniques you use to be personally effective at work or home apply just as much to developing and sustaining you as a leader at work too. These include personal skills such as being assertive, understanding your personality or make-up and exploiting your strengths, realising the causes of stress for you and minimising them and their effects. You will have to be good at prioritising, and brilliant at communicating – to everyone, about everything they need to know to fulfil their role and feel ownership of your organisation at all stages – from early plans to disseminating and celebrating what has been achieved.

Consider what techniques you employ for increasing the efficiency of your work organisation too. If you are to function as an effective leader then you will need to have an efficient and effective work organisation behind you. This will mean reviewing your working practices, systems and procedures. You and your colleagues should not only be well versed in modern theories of management, but able to put them into practice in a coherent way, reviewing progress and overcoming barriers to change, working for consistent improvement.

> Personal and organisational success is heavily dependent on understanding the context and developing successful interpersonal and inter-organisational relationships in order to move forwards with change. Leadership is not a series of single actions but a process of continual interaction with others to influence and persuade ... local managerial reputations are made or lost by tackling big issues that are regarded as important by local stakeholders ... Leadership is after all, about differentiating yourself successfully from the crowd.
>
> Neil Goodwin, Chief Executive,
> Greater Manchester Strategic Health Authority
> HSJ columnist, 2006

Your techniques

Be rightly assertive. As a leader, your biggest challenge may be being assertive with yourself so that you don't agree to take on additional tasks that are not essential for you to undertake, or that fall outside your own priority areas.

Assertiveness is about knowing and practising your rights – to change your mind, to make mistakes, to not understand about something, to refuse demands, to express emotions, to be yourself. As a leader this can be difficult if you are torn between loyalty to the overall organisation and your commitment to your managers, and your own inclinations. There is a narrow line between behaving in an assertive manner, or in an aggressive or bossy way – it takes practice to get it right.

Make effective decisions. Be decisive and finish jobs that you have in hand. Gather information about a problem or choice, be consultative, weigh up the pros and cons and make a decision. Once you have made that decision look forward and make plans for the future. Don't look backwards and frame regrets.

Motivation. Think what your own motives are for assuming your leadership role. The best motivators for fulfilling people's needs are:

- interesting and/or useful work
- a sense of achievement
- responsibility
- opportunities for career progression or professional development
- gaining new skills and competencies
- a sense of belonging (to a professional group, employing organisation or workplace team).

So consider if one or more of these factors drive you on or give you increased job satisfaction.

Control your work flow. Review the flow of your work so that it matches your capacity. You will probably be most productive with a steady flow of work rather than having a 'pressure/slack/pressure' sandwich. Do as many non-urgent jobs as possible in the quieter periods to keep up a steady work flow.

Concentrate on one task at a time. Complete it and either move on to another job or take a short break to refresh yourself and clear your mind so that you are ready to start again. Maintain control of your paperwork. Don't let it build up so that you feel overwhelmed by it. Otherwise you will put off tackling it at all or work more slowly as the enormity of the task depresses you.

Stress management. Stress at work does not happen in a 'vacuum'. Pressures at home often overflow onto how you feel and perform at work, and vice versa. There are three types of responses to stress – physiological, psychological and behavioural reactions. The way you respond depends on personal factors such as your age, gender, personality, previous family and personal experiences, other life events that are happening to you, as well as your coping ability and other organisational options.

The effects of stress in the workplace to watch out for and prevent as a leader, include:

- reduced productivity
- lack of creativity
- increased errors
- poor decision making
- job dissatisfaction
- poor timekeeping

- disloyalty
- increased extent of sick leave
- increased number of complaints
- premature retirement
- absenteeism
- accidents
- theft
- organisational breakdown.

Stress can affect everyone. It often goes undetected or unacknowledged by individuals themselves. They may have been warned by others to 'slow down' and have delighted in ignoring such advice and pushing themselves on regardless. Often people with 'Type A' personalities react like this. Type A behaviour is often learned in childhood, when the child strove to achieve as a way of counteracting their low self-esteem or self-worth. Although some people with Type A characteristics believe they are a positive benefit to help them get through their work quickly, in the longer term these characteristics can be self-destructive. People with Type B personalities can be just as successful and achieve just as much as those with Type A personality types, but at a slower, steady pace. If you recognise yourself as having a Type A personality you can modify your behaviour with practice.

The kind of practical methods you could use to cope with stress at work for yourself are to:

- identify the prime causes of stress or pressure and then make changes to reduce or avoid them
- seek support from colleagues/family/friends
- share problems with suitable colleagues; admit your doubts and worries to others
- adopt better time management practices
- protect time off-duty
- develop a better balance between your work and home commitments
- stop being a perfectionist.

Look after your health. Don't deny your own needs for rest and recuperation. You are not indispensable. Compare how you behave when you are ill with what most people would do and try and narrow the gap. Staying fit and healthy involves a combination of good physical, mental and spiritual wellbeing.

Stay on top to sustain your enthusiasm for learning and your quest for knowledge and understanding. The personal satisfaction that you gain from completing a project, degree or some other educational experience should make you feel more fulfilled and re-awaken your interest in a wide range of practice. Positive thinking and finding time for personal and professional development are vital.

Top tips

Here's a real bonus – two sets of top tips for you.

1 Tips on making effective decisions.
   - There are always other options – find out what they are.
   - Gather ideas and evidence from other people or a range of sources – do not

be confined only to the options you already know about.

- Base your analyses and decisions on reliable objective evidence or observations, and not on 'guesstimates'.
- Think through the implications of your decision by considering the possible consequences before choosing which option to take.
- Information is about feelings as well as facts – how the situation really is and how people feel about it.
- Remember that your personality and beliefs will affect your decision making process.
- Don't accept other people's perceptions of reality – look and think for yourself.
- Be honest with yourself and others, and keep your integrity. The best decisions are based on truth and not illusions.
- Effective decisions are based on reality and not hope.
- Probing questions help to distinguish between illusion and reality.
- Simple decisions are usually best and often obvious in retrospect.
- Fear can get in the way of making realistic assessments of the possible options.

Don't make decisions because you are frightened of something, but because you are enthusiastic about the expected outcomes.

2 Tips for being assertive.
- Say 'NO' clearly and then move away or change the subject. Keep repeating 'NO' – don't be diverted. You don't necessarily need to explain or justify yourself.
- Be honest and direct with everyone.
- Don't apologise or justify yourself more than is reasonable.
- Offer a workable compromise and negotiate an agreement that suits you and the other person.
- Pause before answering a 'YES' you'll regret. Delay your response and give yourself more time to think by asking for more information. So instead say 'Let me think about that'. Think of the cost of saying 'yes' and what you will gain by saying 'no'.
- Keep your body language as assertive as possible. Match your tone to your words (don't smile if you are giving a serious message).
- Use the 'broken record' technique – persistently repeat your message in a calm manner to someone who is trying to pressurise you to do something you don't want to do. Don't be side-tracked.
- Show that you are listening to the other person's point of view and are giving them a fair hearing.
- Practise expressing your opinions and rights rather than expecting other people to guess what you want.
- Don't be too hard on yourself if you make a mistake – everyone is human.
- Be confident enough to change your mind if that is appropriate.
- It can be assertive to say nothing.

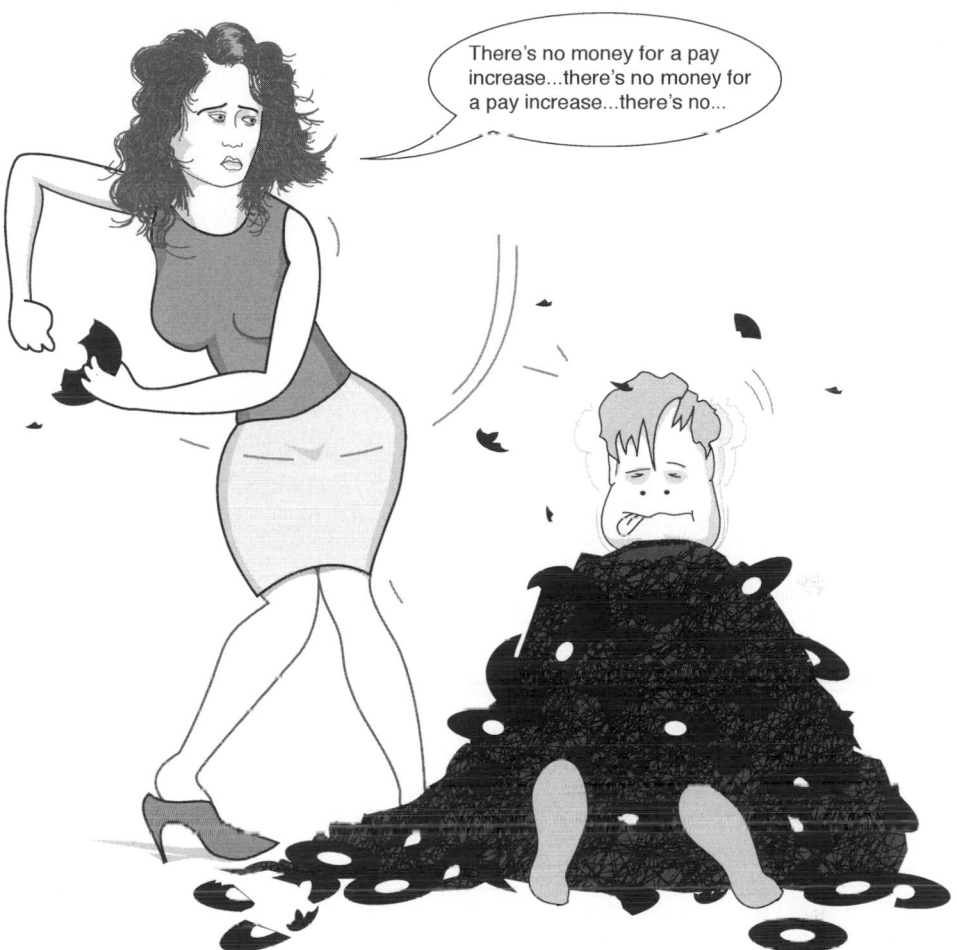

The broken record technique.

Frequently asked questions and answers

Q. *Do you think that as a leader I perform better under pressure, so really in all honesty, stress management is for wimps?*

A. There is a common misconception amongst senior people working in the NHS that there is a linear relationship between the extent of demands on individuals and their performance at work. But actually there is an optimum level of demand where you are decisive, creative, working efficiently and effective. After this point if a sensible level of demand is exceeded, your performance tails off and you become less effective, less decisive etc., and eventually exhausted and burnt out.

Q. *One of the problems with being a leader in the NHS is sustaining strong leadership in circumstances where you have little control, with the various government imperatives raining down on you and rapidly revolving priorities. What can I do to keep control of our work programme for my department?*

A. Review the degree to which you are in control of your work and how much more control you should try to take. Stop banging your head against a brick wall trying to control things that you have no chance of changing. Become more laid back and reserve your energy for being in control of things that really matter. Networking with other leaders in a learner set or at meetings can help as you share experiences and solutions, and provide you with the right kind of support and encouragement.

Interactive exercise: reflect on how effective you are from all angles

Look at how good you are at making effective decisions.

Step 1: think through your general approach to making a decision:
- how good do you think you are in general about making effective decisions?
- what is stopping you from being more decisive?
- how often do you regret a decision that you have made? Is it *often/seldom/never*?
- how often do you ruminate over decisions, thinking over and over again about whether you did the right thing? Is it *often/seldom/never*?

Step 2: now work through a specific example by yourself. Describe an important decision that you have to make now or in the near future to do with your job as a leader:
- what are the options?
- what are the circumstances or potential advantages of your preferred option?
- what are the circumstances or potential disadvantages of your preferred option?
- what other information do you need to find out before making your decision?
- how sure are you that you have all the information possible, and have thought through the consequences of your decision for yourself and their effects on other people?
- if you have decided not to make any decision in the short-term when will you review the situation?

- how much is your decision a positive choice or rather one where you are making the best of things?
- is there any other way that you could be more effective about making this decision?

Step 3: lastly, reflect on what you have written down in the exercise – thinking of how effective you might seem to be to someone else in the organisational hierarchy above you, or a peer or partner if you are already at or near the top of your organisation. Think how effective you would seem to be to someone lower down in the hierarchy, another member of your team, or someone who will be affected by your decision. Then discuss the example you have chosen and worked through and your reflections with someone else whose opinion you value – maybe another leader in a similar position to yourself, or a more experienced leader than you, or your mentor if you have one.

Chapter 5

Competencies of a good leader

Robert Cragg and Peter Spurgeon

Introduction

A competency is a skill that an individual has, which equips them to perform a specific task. Just as a mechanic requires a precise set of skills to mend cars, leaders require a certain array of competencies to enact effective leadership.

Leadership is an often misunderstood, nebulous concept, difficult to define and frequently contested, owing to the diversity of contexts in which leadership can be expressed.[1] As a consequence there are a plethora of models, frameworks and theories to describe leadership in both academic and populist literature.

Leadership traits have developed throughout history linked to emotive religious, political and military icons.[2] In this chapter we consider the development of leadership theory through the 20th century covering the three most commonly referenced theories: *trait theory, situational leadership* and *transformational leadership* – discussing their relative validity and application today. The common thread to these contrasting models is the core concept of leadership as a process of influence.

> The kind of leadership that is required (in the NHS) is transformational leadership.
>
> Alimo-Metcalfe[3]

Main theories and models of leadership

1 Trait theory

Trait theory implies that leaders are born rather than developed, supporting the notion that leaders have an innate superiority that makes them naturally predisposed to positions of importance and power. The theory attempts to characterise the identification of personal attributes that separate leaders from others.[4] This field of research identifies traits such as charisma, courage and intelligence.

Trait theory has been largely disregarded by researchers as providing no tangible basis for leadership development. But, although considered outdated, the traits emerging from this theory still influence the selection of leaders today.[4]

2 Situational leadership

This model claims that it is the situation itself that determines the person who emerges as the leader, so that an individual's competencies and style are complementary to the task. Consequently this theory implies that no one individual is able to lead across all tasks and scenarios, and that a person's leadership potential is narrow and inflexible when the environment changes.[2] A case study alleged to illustrate this notion relates to Winston Churchill's meteoric war time rise and post war slump in popularity with voters, demonstrating that the former prime minister excelled in leading military strategy but failed to retain his followers during the post war hardships, amidst voters' demands for social reforms.

With the situational model is the realisation that leadership is embodied in us all. To achieve the full multifaceted gamut of leadership competencies, you must harness the collective talents of your team, as well as yours as an individual. Organisations should enhance leadership potential in the workforce within team settings, at every level of service.[5] Whilst leaders have a strong preference for one style, the key is to develop flexibility but at the same time acknowledge their own limitations.

3 Transactional and transformational leadership

The transformational model of leadership is synonymous with the proactive implementation of change and the concept of the servant leader.[6] Empowerment is key by which the leader unifies followers through a shared vision, trust and common values, imparting their influence across networks of individuals to deliver service development.[7]

Bass identified key behavioural dimensions including intellectual stimulation through questioning and thinking creatively; these are – consideration, value and development of others.[7] Alimo-Metcalfe and Alban-Metcalfe identified characteristics that staff required of their leaders.[5] They recognised qualities typified by the transformational model including; 'concern for others, approachability, encouraging questioning, promoting change; the ability to communicate, set direction, unify and manage change'.[5] These competencies do not include being brash and overly confident as a stereotyped notion of leaders suggests, but instead emphasise subtlety and imply an emotional intelligence and inquisitive disposition.

By contrast, the transactional model of leadership offers an incentive based exchange between the leader and follower in return for enhanced performance. This approach is task focused, reliant on hierarchy and bypasses the requirement to engage individual principles; thus the process is more short-term.[8] Transactional leadership concerns maintenance and monitoring of a pre-existing service, having an operational rather than a strategic focus.[4,5]

Emergent competencies

The study of leadership theory dispelled the myth that leadership requires superhuman qualities, in favour of a more practical model of leadership which lends itself to development.[1]

The competencies emerging from three of the models (trait theory, transactional and transformational models, *see* Table 5.1) though largely derived from the private sector, resonate within the public sector too including the NHS. Their transferability implies that the skills required for leadership are largely universal, be it in a managerial, professional or political context.[4]

Table 5.1 Comparison of leadership models: as to their qualities, skills and attributes.

Trait theory	Transactional	Transformational
Courage	Making operational	Being visionary
Charisma	decisions	Promoting change
Intelligence	Driving for results	Setting direction
Integrity	Developing teams	Questioning tendency
Self-belief – confidence	Technical awareness	Political astuteness
Self-motivation	Business acumen	Inspiring
Enthusiasm	Holding to account	Making strategic decisions
Self-awareness	Conflict resolution	Driving for improvement
Trust and loyalty	Delegation	Leading change through
Commanding respect	Planning/finance	people
Steadfastness	Performance focused	Innovation/creativity
Role model	Monitoring	Developmental
	Influencing through	Empowering
	incentives	

Leadership frameworks

The diverse range of leadership competency frameworks can be confusing. Which one do you follow? There are the NHS leadership qualities framework,[9] Dye and Garmans' exceptional leadership model,[10] John Adair's task-team-individual model[3] or Alimo-Metcalfe's 21st century model of leadership[1] to name but a few.

The NHS has developed the leadership qualities framework as a guide to the leadership characteristics it feels healthcare workers need to adopt (*see* Table 5.2). The 15 qualities within the framework are grouped in three clusters – personal qualities, setting direction and delivering the service. This framework has been instrumental in establishing leadership development activities across the NHS. (*see* www.nhsleadershipqualities.nhs.uk).[9]

Table 5.2 Leadership qualities framework.

Personal qualities	Setting direction	Delivering the service
Self-belief	Seizing the future	Leading change through
Self-awareness	Intellectual flexibility	people
Self-management	Broad scanning	Holding to account
Drive for improvement	Political astuteness	Empowering others
Personal integrity	Drive for results	Effective and strategic
		influencing
		Collaborative working

Dye and Garmans' model has 16 critical competencies for healthcare executives; it draws out many of the same themes as in the leadership qualities framework centred around the four clusters of: well cultivated self-awareness, compelling vision, masterful execution and real way with people (*see* Table 5.3).[10] Whilst there are countless competency models there is great similarity and overlap between them, as seemingly distinct characteristics of one model are often merely approximate synonyms from another.[3]

Table 5.3 Dye and Garman's model of leadership.

Well cultivated self-awareness	Compelling vision	Masterful execution	Real way with people
Personal conviction Emotional intelligence	Being visionary Communicating vision Earning loyalty and trust	Listening like you mean it Giving feedback Mentoring others Developing teams Energising staff	Generating informal power Building consensus Making decisions Driving results Stimulating creativity Cultivating adaptability

Leadership roles need to be created with reference to a model of effective leadership that the organisation endorses and upholds according to its culture and objectives.

Every employing organisation needs a leadership framework to both select and build capacity for the competencies it requires to achieve success. Competencies must be selected carefully balancing the trade off of a specific versus generic scope, individual versus organisational need, whilst considering the requirement for future adaptivity.[4]

Top tips

- No one leader has the skills, knowledge and behaviour to be effective in all situations.
- Leadership is not a construct reserved for individuals but can be displayed by teams too.
- Organisations should not develop leadership competencies at the expense of management skills.
- Teams need managers to promote stability and leaders to press for change.
- If there is too much transactional management teams stagnate. If there is too much transformational leadership then organisations can become chaotic.[5]
- When you have mapped the leadership competencies in your existing team and people's strengths, use this information to allocate tasks so that you maximise the overall performance of the team. Ask those with the right competencies if they will act as coaches and role models for colleagues wishing to acquire that skill.
- Remember leadership skills can be developed. Just because you don't excel in a given competency today doesn't mean you can't acquire it in the future.
- Reflect on leaders that have influenced you. What qualities did they have that impressed you? Role modelling of this kind can make you more perceptive to behaviours that display effective leadership.
- Leadership models which incorporate both change and the adoption of organisational culture, start to provide a link between leadership performance and organisational success. This can be assessed by the ability of the leader to change individuals to embrace a transformational culture.[1]
- Training and conceptualisation is key to instigate the appropriate cultural context within which leadership can prosper.

- Challenge and responsive feedback along the way ensure that interim and post project evaluations take place to assess the success of both learning and delivery.
- There is no fixed model of leadership to follow; the overriding approach needs to match the individual and the context.

Frequently asked questions and answers

Q. *How can different leadership theories be reconciled and how can we relate leadership competence to performance?*
A. There is a constant tension between leadership where a range of personal characteristics are emphasised, as against the understanding of tasks and behaviours that might constitute leadership. This tension can be reconciled as simple components of the same dynamic theory. The raw ingredients of leadership, your natural innate and acquired competencies (inputs), determine your behaviour in response to specific tasks and leadership situations (enactment). The appropriateness of your behaviour and influence with a given context or situation directly correlates to your performance (outputs) in fulfilling your leadership objectives. Leadership works when it is defined by outcomes.

Q. *How can I develop and learn more about my personal leadership style?*
A. Knowledge of models and traits should be compulsory for prospective and current leaders, teamed with a supportive development pack to improve their skills. You must maximise the enactment of both your innate and acquired competencies, learning to deploy your skills and attributes in a flexible and adaptive manner to be an effective leader. Being aware of your personal competency levels is critical.

Q. *How can I find out more about my strengths and weaknesses?*
A. Self-awareness can be improved through psychometric tests, which should give you insights into your personal preferences, e.g. Myers Briggs (*see* the exercise in Chapter 3 too).

Interactive exercise: gridlocked: analysing your competencies as a leader

You can develop a framework to apply your newfound comprehension of leadership competencies in order to identify the skills that your work role demands. First off is your need to develop more self-awareness in respect of the competencies you currently hold and those that you need to acquire. Combine doing this exercise with the evolution of your personal development plan, to capture your current competencies in leadership as a benchmark on which to build your future development.

Step 1: list the competencies that are pertinent to your current job-role or a specific project on which you are set to embark.

Step 2: place each competency onto a grid similar to that in Table 5.4 according to your previous experience and comfort level. Discuss this part of the exercise with a colleague, mentor or your line manager to consider the differing needs between your competency and that required by the job. Competencies placed in each quadrant will fit the following descriptions.

- Quadrant 1. Tasks involving these competencies may cause you anxiety. You may have previously avoided this type of task. You will need to acquire confidence in enacting this competency.
- Quadrant 2. A competency in this quadrant requires expansion of your current skill set. You may be apprehensive about tasks incorporating this competency, due to the development challenges it poses.
- Quadrant 3. Unchallenging, not stimulating, limited development, 'Been there, done that'.
- Quadrant 4. Provides an easy challenge. Good personal development, increasing your competency portfolio. You are eager to engage with the opportunity.

Table 5.4 Competency grid.

		Competency previously experienced	Competency not previously experienced
LEARNING REQUIRED ↑	Outside comfort zone	Quadrant 1	Quadrant 2
	Inside comfort zone	Quadrant 3	Quadrant 4

Step 3: identify and prioritise goals for developing the competencies identified in Quadrants 1, 2 and 4, accounting for the size of the learning gap you need to overcome. Aim for a good balance of development. If you stay in your comfort zone all the time you will eventually lack flexibility and lose your willingness to accommodate others' styles and acquire new skills. Conversely if you seek to develop yourself too much or too quickly you might become susceptible to stress and find it difficult to cope.

References

1 Alimo-Metcalfe B, Lawler J. Leadership development in UK companies at the beginning of the twenty-first century. Lessons for the NHS? *J Healthc Manag Med.* 2001; **15**(5): 387–404.
2 Olivier R. *Inspirational leadership – Henry V and the muse of fire.* London: Spiro Press; 2001.
3 Alimo-Metcalfe B, Alban-Metcalfe J. Half the battle. *Health Serv J.* 2002; **112**(5795); 26–7.
4 Adair J. *Effective Leadership.* 2nd ed. London: Pan Books Ltd; 1988.
5 Kotter J. *What Leaders Really Do.* Harvard: Harvard Business School Press; 1999.
6 Greenleaf RK. *The Servant Leader Within: a transformative path.* New Jersey: Paulist Press International; 2003.
7 Bass BM. *Leadership and performance beyond expectations.* New York: Free Press; 1985.
8 Turrill T. *Change and innovation: a challenge for the NHS.* Management Series 10. London: Institute of Health Services Management; 1986.

9   NHS Leadership Centre. *Leadership Qualities Framework;* 2002 www.nhsleadership qualities.nhs.uk.

10   Dye CF, Garman AN. *Exceptional Leadership – 16 critical competencies for healthcare executives.* Chicago: Health Administrative Press; 2006.

Chapter 6

Leading the way as a good employer

Ruth Chambers

Introduction

Your greatest asset is your staff. As practices and trusts become larger, good human resources management is essential to the delivery of your care and services. So you will want to select and recruit staff in a fair and equitable way to complement your practice or departmental ethos and match your team's needs.

As the leader you will tackle any discrimination, harassment or bullying in your workplace. You'll know that the quality of the induction you arrange for new staff is an important facet in determining how quickly and safely they become established in any new healthcare setting.

The results of your good employment practices and responsive management will be high standards of performance by happy, well motivated staff. The whole team must function appropriately at all levels for the quality of care and services you provide to be assured. You will design jobs and roles so that people perform well. You will invest time and energy in supporting and listening to people, and know how to motivate people and encourage high standards.

A positive culture and good employment practices will include regular feedback to staff about their performance, clear leadership from you and other leaders at all levels, good communication to everyone about everything. So you will be responsive and as priorities alter, recognise the pressures that people are under when there is uncertainty and change and help them to acclimatise to new ways of working.

> Context is important because it raises the question not of whether leaders make a difference, but more importantly under what conditions they can make a difference.
>
> Neil Goodwin, Chief Executive,
> Greater Manchester Strategic Health Authority
> HSJ columnist, 2006.

Leading the way to good employment practices

Your developmental approach to the staff. Achieving continuous improvement in performance requires that you adopt a developmental approach that encourages staff, rather than issue 'top down' directives that are resented by staff and difficult to implement. So try to include the whole team in discussing the need to make changes and in evolving your plans for change. Listen to and act on their views as far as possible – their frontline perspectives are invaluable in solving problems and improving your systems and processes.

The three components of good organisational management are:

1 people
2 environment
3 process.

People. Consider the number of skilled and experienced staff you will need to deliver your vision of care and services. Concentrate on building up cohesive teams that function effectively under good leadership. Create the environment and processes within your practice or trust that breed well motivated staff with high levels of job satisfaction.

Environment. The environment includes the physical structure of your premises and contents, and the technical capacity such as medical equipment and IT hardware and software. Regular and thorough risk assessment, followed by risk reduction and monitoring are essential aspects of good organisational management of the environment in your workplace. So review what statutory and mandatory training should be in place for your staff; and check your systems for monitoring that staff are attending and/or being assessed as to their knowledge and skills as expected or required.

Process. Process includes policies, procedures and systems. Good organisational management of the process of planning and delivering care and services will reduce the chances of mistakes happening at work. Errors should be picked up by fail-safe systems before there is any opportunity for harm. Good processes will ensure that staff only undertake activities for which they are competent – important when a great deal of training happens in the workplace such as for healthcare assistants who need to be trained and assessed by supervising nurses or allied health professionals (AHPs) before they take on tasks that were previously within the remit of the nurse or AHP. Well-disseminated policies allow everyone in the workplace to know how systems and procedures work and give consistent messages to patients.

Equity is an important end point that can be used as a measure of a good employer.

Equity might concern:

- equal access to opportunities for staff development
- equal treatment about covering least favourite duties, e.g. covering public holidays
- allowances for staff with disabilities, e.g. special chairs
- that staff working in branch surgeries or peripheral clinics are not disadvantaged
- balance and interest of workload between health professionals and managers and other staff
- proportional share of responsibilities
- democratic decision making.

Release others' talents. Identify and overcome barriers for individuals, teams and organisations in achieving their potential. Ensure that individuals' learning and development needs are identified and met. Training for all staff should:

- be based on their personal and professional needs
- be available to all in an equitable way depending on professional and service needs
- reflect multidisciplinary working
- be delivered or available in an appropriate format for what they need to learn (e.g. e-learning, plenary presentations, small group work, reading and reflecting).

Appraisal. Good employment practice includes regular job appraisal, at least annually. This gives individuals an opportunity to review how well they are doing in their own view and that of the person who is appraising them. Employed staff can agree learning needs and how they will be met in the context of their current job or agreed changes to their roles and responsibilities.

Under-performance can cover a range of issues such as people's knowledge, skills, behaviour and attitudes. As a leader you will have to create or oversee systems to diagnose, assess and support those for whom you are responsible who may be under-performing. Under-performance is about achieving less than expected, or performing below required levels or explicit standards. Sometimes under-performance is defined in terms of consistently placing patients or others at risk. A single incident will not normally constitute under-performance but repeated less important infringements may. Sometimes the issue is about the work environment or culture leading to a lack of performance, rather than a deficit in someone's knowledge or skills or application.

Individuals who under-perform may:

- be generally passive
- find challenge frightening and avoid it whenever possible
- lack insight about their shortcomings
- find feedback and criticism threatening
- have low reserves of energy
- have poor motivation
- resent others' success
- fail to realise their potential
- be part of a dysfunctional team.

Sometimes the problem arises from a malfunctioning organisation such as:

- poor management of quality processes
- inadequate infrastructure and insufficient resources to undertake tasks
- poor communication within the work setting
- an unhealthy culture within the organisation
- a culture of fear and lack of openness
- a lack of leadership, or inappropriate style of management or poor organisational structure.

Top tips

- Investigate cases of possible under-performance within well defined timescales in a proper way: specific to the individual concerned and the area of concern, with measures based on agreed indicators that are clear, simple and understood.

- In proven cases of under-performance: consider providing support through mentorship; assess training and development needs; agree a programme to meet these needs; agree short-term action plans with performance targets. Think more widely about the relevance of a programme to build the individual's self-esteem or develop their assertiveness skills, providing training to change their attitudes, or changing the environment to suit the needs of the individual. Use formal disciplinary measures as a last resort or reserve them for serious cases.
- Develop skills in delegating and trusting people to attend to the detail while you keep to the overall direction.
- Set out the ultimate and intermediate goals for your team; don't drift along as that reduces motivation and drive.
- Ensure that everyone is well informed about any employment issues. Squash unsubstantiated rumours so that they do not unsettle people.
- Try new ways of coping with change and your new circumstances so that the team learns fresh ways of functioning.
- Be available to colleagues, your team and other staff. Some people need little support or supervision. Others need a lot, particularly when they are new to an organisation.
- Acknowledge and praise people's achievements. If all you do is pile on more work, people will become demotivated.
- Resist going for the quick fix rather than understanding and finding solutions that will work in the longer term. The immediate and obvious solution is often wrong because the implications of that change have not been thought through. Further changes are then necessary and people start to doubt that anything will improve.
- Establish good relationships with your team and others so that people feel that they can bring problems to your attention without fear of blame or giving offence.
- Maintain high standards of ethical behaviour, e.g. giving factual, true references; noting, investigating and addressing other people's unacceptable performance or behaviour; or being honest and transparent in financial dealings.
- Encourage a culture where creativity and innovation are welcomed and people learn from past successes and failures.

Frequently asked questions and answers

Q. *My team are pretty confused by all the changes in the health service and concerned that their previous work in planning new services has been wasted. What can I do to help them?*
A. As the leader you should understand the rationale for your practice's or trust's vision – or that of the NHS in general, be able to articulate it and show your staff how the vision can be realised. Then you'll be able to engage people in developing the vision and reflect that vision in your strategies and action plans. Everyone working in your practice or unit should be clear about their goals, roles and responsibilities, the timetables of programmes for improvements, and the standards of performance required of them. With that sort of surety they will be able to progress.

Q. *You talk of allocating funds and opportunities for learning in an equitable way. But that doesn't happen in real life does it when the more powerful professions like doctors dominate and scoop training funds for themselves at the expense of others. Is that fair?*

A. The way that training funds are allocated in your organisation should be an open and transparent process. Allocations should be based on an overview of all staff's training needs; priorities are going to be matched to service needs and professional requirements so that you can provide a safe and effective service for patients. The relative costs of training various types of staff and the nature of what mode of learning they need will all be factors to be considered in dividing up training funds. An organisational policy might specify what proportions of training costs or work/personal time should be covered by the recipient. That proportion might relate to the extent to which training is imperative for the organisation or results in knowledge and skills that are transferable and useful for someone's career progression.

Interactive exercise: listening but not hearing

One of the most common complaints of individuals who are diagnosed as underperforming is that their seniors do not listen to their concerns. This exercise demonstrates the effects of not listening and provides a practical method to improve your listening skills.

You will have to undertake this exercise with another person, or do the exercise with a group of people. You can explore the feelings generated by not listening to someone and demonstrate the powerful technique of 'mirroring' where you actively mirror someone else's body language, eye contact, tone of voice, types of words used and even breathing.

Let's call you person A and the person with whom you are working on this exercise is person B. You as person A sit opposite person B and describe your last major holiday to them in no more than five minutes. Your partner, B, should actively try not to hear what you are saying. They can do anything except leave the chair and make it obvious that they are not 'hearing' you. They should wriggle in the chair, pick up a book and thumb through it, hum, look away at another part of the room.

After five minutes you as person A should repeat your holiday story again to your partner. This time person B should mirror your body language and actively listen to what you are saying. Your partner, B, should respond in the same tone of voice as you're using, copy your posture, maintain eye contact etc.

Then you can both switch roles and your partner B will tell you about their holiday, first without you paying any attention and then with you mirroring them in the same way as described.

Finally you should discuss what feelings were generated by you or your partner in the first half of the exercise compared with when you were individually mirroring each other in turn. If you can see the benefits of this exercise, practise mirroring and active listening in your everyday working life.

Chapter 7

Team leadership

Hugh Flanagan and Veronica Wilkie

Introduction

Working with others has long been recognised as an important feature of delivering patient care. In 1985, the Royal College of General Practitioners recommended that primary care professionals should work more closely together, pooling their skills to improve patient care and enhancing their personal job satisfaction. In 1987, the Health Education Authority introduced a team building training programme for primary care professionals. Since then belief in the importance of team working skills to the success of healthcare delivery in the NHS has continued to grow.[1]

There is evidence that multidisciplinary teamwork in primary care leads to reported improvements in health delivery and staff motivation.[2] But less than one in four healthcare teams have effective communication and team working practices.[3]

Work with a large number of NHS teams in a variety of settings has shown that group processes, communication, clarity of objectives and leadership all enhance team effectiveness as well as promoting good mental health of those working in effective teams.[4]

> Being a part of this team for the last year gave me the greatest learning of my professional career ... I am now learning all over again having become the official leader of the team ...
> (Psychiatrist working with community mental health team)

Team leadership

What is 'a team'? A team can be defined as:

> ... a distinguishable set of two or more people who interact dynamically, interdependently, and adaptively towards a common and valued goal/objective/mission, who each have been assigned specific roles or functions to perform, and who have a limited life-span of membership.'[5]

In a similar vein, others suggest that a team is:

> ... a small number of people with complementary skills who are committed to a common purpose, performance goals, and approach for which they hold themselves mutually accountable.[6]

Teams are distinguished by the degree to which members work in a closely integrated way and/or in geographical proximity to each other, e.g. the close knit operating theatre teams or resuscitation teams versus the more disparate community mental health or midwifery teams.

A 'meeting' is not a team but a means by which teams or representatives from different teams communicate and do business. A team meeting is a good place to observe the culture and characteristics of teams.

The essence of teamworking = task + process. The *task* is derived from an organisational or service context and dictates what process(es) team members need to fulfil to complete the task. *Process* is the mix of practical systems and methods used to get the job done plus team maintenance, i.e. what the team does to raise its performance and develop the skills and motivation of its members to interact effectively.

Task related processes include:

- clarifying your purpose and objectives
- information sharing and use
- decision taking
- methods of communication – within the team and between the team and its wider constituency
- the conduct of team meetings – agenda setting, time-keeping and participation.

Maintenance related process issues include:

- how the team exercises leadership
- how individuals contribute to the team – their professional role/knowledge and their style/behaviour
- how members interact to achieve the task – do they feel part of the team and able to give of their best?

Team maintenance. Teams do not always give attention to how they work, particularly if things seem to be going generally okay. Numerous studies have highlighted the importance of a team climate which is characterised by interpersonal trust and mutual respect, where team members are comfortable being themselves and are confident that they will not be embarrassed, rejected or punished for behaviours such as airing differences or handling confrontations. Both the quality and quantity of team communication appears to be determined by these issues of psychological safety.[7]

Team development theory is concerned with describing the social processes that naturally occur when individuals work together. These may be seen as stages of group development where teams develop through a set of phases,[8,9] i.e:

- forming – the group comes together and the predominant concerns are those of acceptance and place in the group, rather than the purpose and tasks of the team. At this stage leadership needs to be specific and directive of the process. The task is defined by the leader
- storming – not necessarily overt conflict but a process of 'sorting out' task and process issues – clarifying 'tasks' and testing the 'process'. The leader needs to allow and encourage exploration and questioning in this adolescent stage
- norming – ways of working that seem to be effective become established. Team members understand the task and their contribution and have a sufficient

degree of trust to communicate effectively. Leadership can now be less directive and more enabling

- performing – the mature team is working and this builds on the successful achievement of the task. Leadership becomes more facilitative and shared.

Teams need to be self-aware of their stage of development. The process of becoming a mature and effective team can be accelerated through regular review and reflection and by taking the necessary maintenance and development actions. A significant change in the internal or external context of the team may affect the performance of even a mature, well-performing team, e.g. a major change in policy, an alteration in the priority of a task of the team or having a new team member – all require proactive consideration and incorporation.

Despite the assumption that pooling of expertise should automatically result in enhanced performance, interdisciplinary teams do not always work well in practice.[10] Interpersonal conflict, communication blocks, low morale and poor performance frequently blight these teams. Teams have to work at becoming and staying effective.

Team decision making. A key feature of everyday teamwork is decision making. So what method is appropriate to the task of the team? Teams need to decide how they will make decisions in the variety of circumstances that the team and its individual members will encounter, e.g. deciding how decisions will be made in certain critical or emergency situations that they anticipate.

Observing team meetings is a good way of identifying the overall cultural 'norm' of the team in decision-taking, e.g:

- lack of response: the 'plop' or lead balloon approach where no one responds to, or builds on, ideas because of their lack of motivation or absence of active listening
- authority rule: the person in the chair makes the decisions – which might be a substitute for personal commitment by team members or the preferred style of the chair
- minority rule: railroading, intimidating, fixing – where the team is not particularly cohesive and different factions and individuals are intent on pursuing their own agendas
- majority rule: voting/polling – which might be an illustration of efficient democracy, or laziness or avoidance of differences
- consensus: everyone has their say, differences are seen as helpful and worked through, decisions are reached which hold up under external scrutiny. This is probably the most effective general approach but requires focused and efficient teamworking and trust
- unanimity: 'group-think' – can be the result of well-developed teamworking and shared values or a lack of objectivity and challenge.

Team roles – being an effective team member

Much of the current thinking about how to be an effective team member centres on the idea of preferred team roles. A major influence and probably one of the best known, is the description by Belbin that differentiates team roles from work roles.[11,12]

Your work role is defined as 'the mix of tasks and responsibilities undertaken by individuals or within a team'. Your team role is the 'tendency to behave, contribute and interrelate with others in a particular way'. These are described in Table 7.1 with their potential contributions to the overall team along with the possible weaknesses that individual team member types may have.

Table 7.1 Potential contributions to the team by individual team types.[12]

Team role	Contribution to the team	Allowable weaknesses
Plant	Creative, solves difficult problems, independent outlook	Loses touch with everyday realities?
Resource investigator	Enterprising, quick to explore new opportunities	Weak in follow through?
Coordinator/ chair	Makes good use of group activities and team members, good communicator	Manipulative?
Shaper	Thrusting, challenging, pushes group	Provocative, aggressive, intolerant?
Monitor/ evaluator	Critical thinking ability, discerning, objective	Hypercritical, uninspiring, sceptical?
Team worker	Cooperative, averts friction, aware of underlying feelings in team	Indecisive?
Implementer/ company worker	Organised, efficient, practical	Slow to see new possibilities?
Completer/ finisher	Painstaking, conscientious, aware of deadlines	Anxious, reluctant to delegate?

Another fairly well known approach is the 'Management Team Wheel' which describes alternative roles, i.e. Explorer/Promoter, Assessor/Developer, Thruster/Organiser, Concluder/Producer, Controller/Inspector, Upholder/ Maintainer, Reporter/Adviser and Creator/Innovator.[13]

Both the Belbin,[12] and Margerison and McCann[13] approaches invite individuals to express their preferences for particular team roles. This is on the basis that a person will contribute to the team in their preferred role at an enhanced level compared to being forced to participate in a less-preferred role. The underlying model is that a team needs all of the roles in order to function effectively and that an absence or imbalance of team member types will lead to less than optimal functioning of the team.

Top tips

1 On being the leader. To maximise your effective leadership of teams:
   - ensure clarity of purpose, context and specific tasks – yours and the team's
   - communicate this constantly within the team and between the team and the rest of the organisation
   - know your team members and when you need to adapt your approach
   - balance directing with empowering the team
   - ensure review and reflection on performance for all team members

- give time and attention to developing the team
- provide support whilst challenging individual members of the team in order to ensure that different views get heard.

2 On being 'a player'. To maximise being an effective player in the team:
- ensure that you understand the purpose, context and specific tasks of the team
- know and communicate your role and particular contribution to others within and outside the team
- contribute proactively and enable others to do the same
- take your share of responsibility for team performance and development
- participate in review, reflection and development
- support colleagues and view different ideas and opinions as initially helpful.

Frequently asked questions and answers

Q. *When do you need a team?*
A. The requirement for a 'team' depends on a number of factors including the complexity of the task, the need for the integration of multiple skills and knowledge within the team such as speed – as in emergency situations, high volume, tight timescales or social isolation.

Q. *What makes teams effective?*
A. Teams don't just happen. You have to work at building and maintaining a team. This requires an understanding of both the task and process issues. Tasks may change and evolve over time. Processes need to be appropriate to the task. Ultimately the team must maintain and develop itself as an effective human group. The organisational context in which teams operate may have as much to do with their success as their internal operations, i.e. consider the extent to which the context actually facilitates and rewards teamworking.

Interactive exercise: team development and expectations

You might organise this exercise as team leader for a newly formed team, or one that is undertaking a review of its effectiveness. The exercise is about clarifying what team members expect or need from each other in the context of maximising the performance of the team. It raises questions about individuals' roles, communication and contributions and the underlying or implicit assumptions you may be making about other team members. It is based on the original work of John Machin in relation to expectations analysis.[14]

Essentially you will organise a series of discussions between paired members of the team to establish what they expect from each other. In the example we have person A and person B.

Prior to meeting, each person prepares for the exercise by answering the two questions stated below; with A preparing in relation to B and B preparing in relation to A. Both record their answers.

1 What do I expect from you?
2 What do I think you expect from me?

This can be based on a checklist describing role, information, communication, challenge etc. or left as an open question – all depending on what seems to best meet the needs of the team and the underlying purpose of the exercise.

During the meeting of A and B, decide who will go first – flip a coin or think of a similar way of deciding. To illustrate where A goes first:

- A shares with B the content of 'What do I expect from you?'
- B listens carefully and notes any differences between what A says and their own assumptions about what A expects from them
- A then shares with B the content of 'What do I think you expect from me?'
- B listens carefully and notes any differences between what A says and what they (B) did expect of A
- this is then repeated with B taking the lead and A listening and noting and contrasting. There may be a tendency for B to start commenting on or editing their original expectations of A in the light of what A has said but the exercise works much better if B acts as if they were in fact the first person to speak (although they spoke second). This gives A a much clearer understanding of B's expectations
- each should then take five minutes to review their notes and collect their thoughts
- there then follows a process of sharing and clarifying differences in reverse order to the start, e.g. B now kicks off
- at the end of this exercise the two team members should have a much greater understanding of:
  - how they can best interact and support each other
  - some points for further action by themselves or to share with the team.

The exercise can then be repeated in relation to other team members until all team members have had this dialogue with each other. The team leader or facilitator will need to collate any common issues for the team.

Some practical points:

- in agreeing to undertake this exercise, team members may wish to establish some ground rules
- where there are already relationship issues in the team there must be a consensus on the use of the exercise – consider using a facilitator
- to save time pairs may exchange notes prior to meeting but this requires that careful thought is given to what is being written.

References

1 Cook R. Paths to effective teamwork in primary care settings. *Nursing Times*. 1996; **92**(14): 44–5.
2 Wood N, Farrow S, Elliott B. A review of Primary Health Care Organisations. *J Clin Nurs*. 1994; **3**(4): 243–50.
3 West MA, Slater JA. *The Effectiveness of Team Working in Primary Care*. London: Health Education Authority; 1996.
4 Borrill CS, West M, Shapiro D, *et al*. Team Working and Effectiveness in Health Care. *Brit J Health Care Manag*. 2000; **6**(8): 364–71.
5 Salas E, Dickinson TL, Converse SA, *et al*. Towards an understanding of team performance and training. In: Swezey RW, Salas E, editors. *Teams: their training and performance*. Norwood, NJ: Ablex. Publishing Corporation 1992; 3–29.
6 Katzenback JR, Smith DX. *The Wisdom of Teams*. New York: McKinsey and Company; 1993.

7   Dyer WG. *Team Building: Current Issues and New Alternatives*. Wokingham: Addison-Wesley; 1999.

8   Tuckman BW. Developmental sequence in small groups. *Psychol Bull*. 1965; **63**: 384–99.

9   Tuckman BW, Jensen MA. Stages of Small Groups Revisited. *Group Organ Stud*. 1977; **2**(4): 419–27.

10 Farrell MP, Schmitt MH, Heinneman GD. Informal Roles and the stages of interdisciplinary team development. *Journal of Interprof Care*. 2001; **15**(3): 281–95.

11 Belbin RM. *Management Teams*. New York: John Wiley and Sons; 1981.

12 Belbin RM. *Team Roles at Work*. Oxford: Butterworth-Heinneman Ltd; 1993.

13 Margerison CJ, McCann DJ. *Team Management: practical new approaches*. London: Mercury Business Guides; 1995.

14 Machin J. *Expectations Approach: improving managerial communications and performance*. Maidenhead, Berks: McGraw Hill Education; 1981.

Chapter 8

Change management

Kay Mohanna

Introduction

You live and work in an environment where things are in an almost constant state of change. At the level of organisational or strategic development this is visible and often challenging. But change is also the way you gather new knowledge and skills and develop your beliefs and attitudes. Understanding change is an important part of professional practice. Working as a member of a team often means guiding, supporting or leading people through a process of change, which may be difficult.

Being a leader requires skills in three main areas if you are to be effective in bringing about change:

- understanding barriers
- enabling transition
- sustaining developments.

> Change is not made without inconvenience, even from worse to better.
>
> Johnson, 1755[1]

What makes effective change management?

- **Understanding and overcoming barriers**
  Potential barriers to implementing change need to be identified and clarified before they can be overcome. One of the effects of coming up against barriers to change is to force you to stop and think about what you are trying to achieve. It may be that if you are hitting a brick wall in implementing your strategy there is a reason for this that you should address – to do with you as the leader, your team or the idea. Barriers will affect your progress as a leader as well as that of your team members. These can be personal or organisational barriers and can arise out of motivational, attitudinal or practical logistical difficulties. Not all will be within your capacity to change and you might need to work around such barriers, recruiting support from other team members.
- **Enabling transition**
  A transition phase in any time of change needs skilful leadership. Old and new policies may temporarily co-exist leading to possible confusion. Team members will be on learning curves at different stages of their development and will need time to adjust. Patience may be needed if good ideas are to come to

fruition and a good leader can steady the hand of those ready to pronounce prematurely that a change is 'not working'.

● **Sustaining developments**
Once a change has become the new 'norm' there is a phase before the recent change becomes a non-issue. Leaders need to reinforce policy with mild prompts and reminders. If change is proving painful, the benefits ensuing may need to be reiterated. You need to identify and record success in order to highlight it. In addition there is always the need to evaluate changes and feed back on progress, or introduce further changes to keep the progress on track.

Adopting changes

Everyone in an organisation will not embrace change at the same time or with the same enthusiasm. According to Everett Rogers, people adopt innovations according to the various stages of a normal, bell-shaped curve that you can plot as change 'diffuses' into an organisation (*see* Figure 8.1).[2]

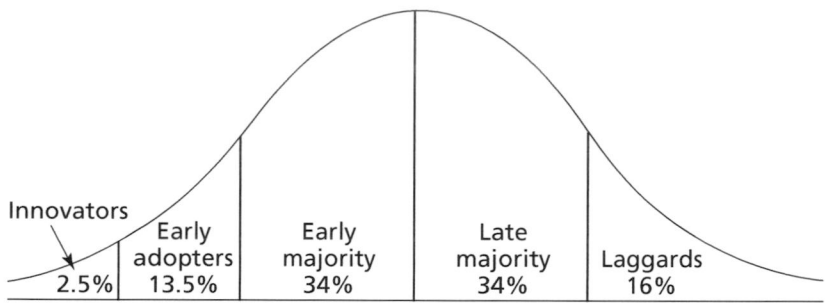

Figure 8.1 Diffusion of innovation.

In Rogers' model, the 'innovators' are the first 2.5% of the people in the organisation to adopt an idea. The next 13.5% to adopt the new idea are the 'early adopters'. The next 34% of the adopters are called the 'early majority'. The 'late majority' are the next 34% to embrace the innovation, and the last 16% to adopt the idea are termed 'laggards'.

It is very important that leaders focus their time and energy appropriately with each particular group of people in bringing about organisational change. In addition, by identifying such team members, leaders can detect, promote or monitor the likelihood of change occurring in an organisation.

● **Innovators**
Innovators are daring, rash and risky. They are able to cope with a high level of uncertainty, but may be considered 'fly by nights' or 'dilettantes'. Rogers says,

> While an innovator may not be respected by the other members of a local system, the innovator plays an important role in the diffusion process; that of launching the new idea in the system by importing the innovation from outside of the system's boundaries. Thus the innovator plays a gatekeeping role in the flow of new ideas into a system.[2]

- **Early adopters**

  Early adopters tend to be opinion leaders. They often serve as role models for other people. They are more integrated into teams than the innovators.

  > The early adopter is respected by his or her peers, and is the embodiment of successful use of new ideas. The early adopter knows that to continue to earn this esteem of colleagues and to maintain a central position in the communication networks of the system, he or she must make judicious innovation-decisions. The early adopter decreases uncertainty about a new idea by adopting it, and then conveying a subjective evaluation of the innovation to peers through interpersonal networks.[2]

- **Early majority**

  The early majority adopts new ideas just before the average member of a system does.

  > The early majority may deliberate for some time before completely adopting a new idea. Their innovation-decision period is relatively longer than that of the innovator and the early adopter. They follow with deliberate willingness in adopting innovations, but seldom lead.[2]

- **Late majority**

  The late majority adopts new ideas just after the average member of a system does. Adoption may be both an economic necessity for the late majority, and the result of increasing network pressures from peers.

  > Innovations are approached with a sceptical and cautious air, and the late majority do not adopt (a change) until most others in their system have done so. The weight of system norms must definitely favour an innovation before the late majority are convinced. The pressure of peers is necessary to motivate adoption.[2]

- **Laggards**

  Laggards are the last in a social system to adopt an innovation. They almost never act as opinion leaders.

  > Laggards tend to be suspicious of innovations and change agents. Their innovation-decision process is relatively lengthy, with adoption and use lagging far behind awareness-knowledge of a new idea. Resistance to innovations on the part of laggards may be entirely rational from the laggards' viewpoint, as their resources are limited and they must be certain that a new idea will not fail before they can adopt it.[2]

Rogers' model is a helpful way of looking at the personalities of team members as it influences their receptiveness to change. Another important factor in whether a change will be adopted is to do with the idea or innovation itself.

The transtheoretical model of the stages of change describes five stages in the adoption of an idea:[3]

- precontemplation
- contemplation
- preparation

- action
- maintenance.

The processes of change may develop through these five stages in order, or in a series of loops as group members confront barriers and rise to the challenges. Any later stage can move to any former stage and these stages may be transient (lasting for minutes or days only). Such swings are a normal part of change.

These stages are often represented as a cycle (*see* Figure 8.2). Members of a group can be at any of these stages at the same time and individual members of the group or team are likely to be at different stages at different times.

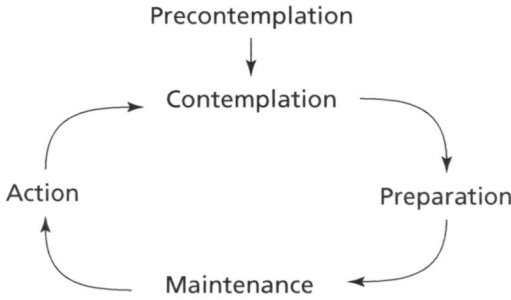

Figure 8.2 Cycle of change.

- **Precontemplation**. Team members or individuals at this stage show no intention to make a change. This is like the teenage smoker who has not even thought that he or she wants to give up. It is just not an issue. It might be because they are busy keeping up with day to day work without stopping to think about change. They may be happy as things are or unaware of different ways to do things.

  One important reason for being stuck at the precontemplative stage of change is when an individual is in a state of 'learned helplessness'. This develops when earlier attempts at implementing change have not been a success, have met with resistance or failed to be maintained. Leaders can suffer from this if they have been discouraged by barriers to change. Team members can suffer from this if organisations do not appear to listen or respond positively to suggestions for change, or if they feel that change is something 'done to them' from outside.

- **Contemplation**. Teams at this stage have begun to think about taking action to implement a change. Self-assessment exercises, audits, critical events or significant event monitoring, or policy changes can all identify areas that might need to be addressed. If proposed changes are in response to a need the team has identified for itself, this stage can be a vigorous phase of discussion and investigation of options. Third party agendas may be met with some ambivalence. 'Chronic contemplators' can make a powerful contribution to a pre-change debate but sometimes need kick-starting by the leader to actually take the first steps. They may be able to identify many potential pitfalls or barriers, thus helping prevent problems before they arise, but this may also paralyse them and inhibit them from action.

Good leaders recognise the roles that people play in response to change:
– the rebel – 'I don't see why I should'
– the victim – 'I suppose you will make me, but I will drag my feet'
– the oppressor – 'You all have to do it'
– the rescuer – 'I will save you all from this terrible change'.

- **Preparation**. There comes a stage when firm plans have to be put in place. Our teenage smoker sets a date to quit, the chronic contemplator has agreed to give it a go and see what happens. If there has been a discussion exercise a decision must be made and leadership skills will be needed to guide the group from their wide ranging discussions to a focused action plan.

  Teams at the preparation stage may have made recent attempts to implement change or carried out small scale or pilot projects. Good leaders will carefully evaluate such attempts and use the findings to guide further planning.

- **Action**. What happens when a new policy is devised, agreed and needs to be implemented? If this results in an overt change in policy, alternative behaviours must be cultivated and old cues and triggers avoided. Smokers who successfully give up, develop alternative activities to do with their hands, avoid those situations where they automatically reach for a cigarette and try not to go to the coffee room or the pub with other smokers.

  There may be some 'grief' issues within the team over the loss of familiar activities and their well established comfort processes. The leader will need to be on the look out for this and combat it in case it threatens to derail progress. This may be simple grumbles or active sabotage.

  Of course the change might not work. All changes must be evaluated. Good leaders use wide ranging methods to gather information about the success of policy change. They talk to all the key players and use objective measures of performance. They will have a contingency management strategy built into the plan.

- **Maintenance**. Good teams, supported by effective leaders, are often rewarded by the successful implementation of new policies. Over time new behaviours are sustained, alternative protocols become established and, later, the fact that there has been a change becomes a non-issue. It is important at this stage that leaders fully evaluate new policies, identify and record success, to build confidence that such challenges can be met in the future.

- **Termination**. The cycle of change never really stops turning in a well managed team, but for each implemented action plan there comes a point when change is sustainable. Earlier policies are not reverted to and the change has been fully incorporated into day to day activity. The leader can then take both eyes off the project and turn their attention to the next challenge.

  We know that people are more likely to be motivated to make a change if:
  – the change is simple
  – it shows an advantage over existing practice
  – it can be tried in practice and seen to work
  – it fits with other areas of established practice
  – personal, professional, social and cultural factors are taken into account.

Top tips

At times of change, good leaders:

- explain why change is needed
- plan for more resources and time than they expect to use, allowing for the unexpected
- consult with team members to understand barriers to the change
- recruit support at the planning stage from 'early adopters'
- beware too many changes taking place at once
- recognise that change can be hijacked by vested interests
- are prepared to change direction if necessary
- facilitate collaboration between team members
- follow up decisions with firm, staged action plans
- fix interval markers of progress
- build in reinforcements and reminders of the new changes and avoidance of old cues and triggers
- have a 'Plan B' for contingency management.

Frequently asked questions and answers

Q. *Help! I have recently taken over as practice manager in a small practice. The doctor wants me to 'update' things but the receptionists have been there for a long time and cannot see the need to change the way they have always done things.*
A. Your staff are at the precontemplation stage and the motivational approach required will be to involve them in suggested changes and raise their awareness of how things could be done or are done elsewhere. Consider a reward system for suggestions that lead to successful changes. Have you got a practice email system or could you start a newsletter with regular updates or meetings to open up the lines of communication? Perhaps there are one or two staff who are a bit more open to new ideas. Could you recruit them to help you?

Q. *What can I do when one team member constantly undermines any suggestions I make?*
A. Why does he or she feel the need to act like this? Is he or she simply a chronic contemplator, potentially full of good ideas and insight into the problems, who is threatened by the idea of change and just needs a gentle nudge to give it a go? Or is it more worryingly a symptom of 'learned helplessness'; that they have had earlier suggestions for change ignored or ridiculed or been involved in changes that did not work? Try involving them, asking for and implementing some of their ideas then providing feedback and encouragement. You may have to design or manipulate the environment to promote success, implement small easily managed changes and provide extra initial resources so that their projects work and you build their confidence.

Interactive exercise: if at first you do not succeed …

When were you last involved with a successful change? Try to fill in all the boxes below. Then try it again for a change that did not work. Reflect on what this shows you about leadership at times of change.

Table 8.1 Reflecting on previous changes.

	A change that worked	*A change that did not work*	*Implication for leadership*
Whose idea was it?			
How much notice did the organisation get of the change?			
How involved was the organisation in planning the change?			
What were the rewards for successful implementation?			
Who bore the costs of implementation?			

References

1   Johnson S. Dictionary of the English Language. (Preface). 1755.
2   Rogers EM. *Diffusion of Innovations*. 4th ed. New York: The Free Press, Simon and Schuster Inc; 1995.
3   Procheska J, Norcross J, DiClemente C. *Changing for Good*. New York: Indigo; 1994.

Chapter 9

Finding time to be a leader

Ruth Chambers

Introduction

As a leader remember that one of the most common sources of stress for you, and your staff and colleagues, is undue time pressure. You need to learn to practise time management unconsciously so that you have sufficient time to invest in being an effective leader. You need to review your priorities and re-allocate the proportions of time you spend on different activities accordingly.

Being good with time is being smarter about getting through your work. A certain degree of time pressure is probably necessary for you to maintain your interest and momentum in getting a job done. Professionals working in the health service are conditioned by their training and the culture at work to feel that they must cope, despite time pressures. They feel that patients must not suffer, whatever the costs to themselves. But there are limits to your tolerance, and if too much pressure is exerted in this way for too long a time, you may end up feeling burnt out and consider leaving your job or profession. So you must learn to control the demands on your time, before any excessive pressures affect you and your performance adversely.

> It enabled me to use time at work effectively.
>
> I have a better insight into how I get distracted by other members of staff and unimportant jobs at work.
>
> I get more done by prioritising the jobs better. I even go home on time these days.
>
> (Pertinent quotes from delegates who undertook a time management workshop.)

Key to good time management

Prioritise your time – do not allow yourself or others to waste it. Be clear about your goals in your work and home lives, or leisure. How you allot your time will look very different if your main goal is to be an international research lead, or learn a new skill such as aromatherapy or nurse prescribing, or to spend as much time as possible with your family. Plan your goals in association with whoever else they affect, and make sure that multiple goals don't conflict with each other.

Spend your 'quality' time doing the most important or complex jobs. It is too easy to focus on getting small unimportant tasks done whilst ignoring the big ones, which just hang over you. A high priority task has to be done, a medium

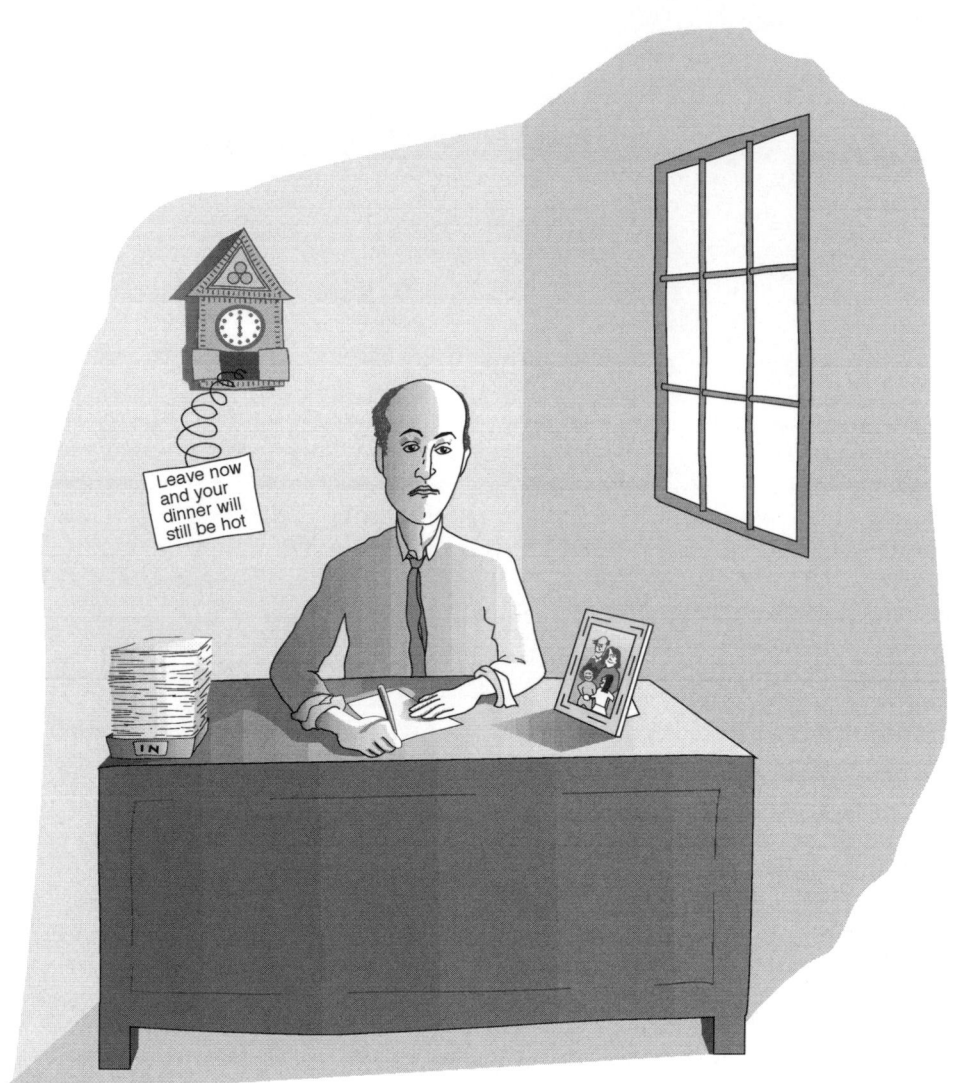

priority job might be delegated, and a low priority task should only be done if you have no medium or high priority tasks waiting, or you are too jaded to tackle them. Don't delay – get on with essential tasks. Distasteful or complicated tasks are the ones that people tend to procrastinate over. If you procrastinate too long the job will be even more difficult, as you will forget your previous ideas or what the instructions were. If you train yourself to do the least wanted task first you can reward yourself with a more pleasing job or even enjoying some free time.

You will achieve more in designated sessions of quiet uninterrupted periods than in a longer allotment of time broken up by various activities. This is the time for planning, writing reports, or analysing progress.

Interruptions are one of the biggest timewasters, especially if someone else could have handled the problem or taken the message, or no action was required. Even if an interruption is necessary it may occur at the wrong time wrecking your concentration or train of thought. Agree rules in your workplace for who may be interrupted and when. Work out a system (and keep to it!) with your colleagues and others at work for letting others know when you are not to be disturbed and are spending quality time on priority tasks, and when you are available to deal with the queries that have built up whilst you were occupied. Keep focused on your priorities and don't allow others to engage you in chat when you are intent on work. Get into the habit of regarding minutes or hours as costed time – think of the worth of some of the activities on which you spend time, and whether different activities are of equal weight.

Include sufficient time for thinking, doing, meeting, developing and learning. You need to be fresh and creative to stay on top of the demands made on you as a leader so that you remain productive. You can only manage this in the longer term if you timetable the right mix of stimulating work, personal and professional development and networking into your daily schedule.

You will have your own preference for ensuring thinking time, which to some extent will depend on your personality. Extroverts will be revitalised by brainstorming and discussions with others, whilst those who are more introverted will prefer protected space in which to reflect and read by themselves. Whichever you prefer make sure you get enough of it to replenish your creativity and enthusiasm.

Try to allow at least 10% of your time for dealing with unexpected tasks. Being a leader invariably means that you will have unexpected work to do and pressing issues to resolve. In the unlikely event that everything goes smoothly and you do not need the extra time, it will be a bonus to have that additional space to catch up on your paperwork, or simply spend a little more time talking to patients and/or colleagues about how they are feeling.

Delegate whatever and however you can; try only to accept delegated work without further training if you have the necessary skills, time and experience. There is a great potential for time wasting if you try and carry out delegated work when you don't know what is required or how to set about doing it. If you are in a position to delegate work and responsibilities, decide what only YOU can do and delegate as much as possible of the rest to others. It is important to reduce duplication as much as possible so that work and initiatives are coordinated throughout your organisation.

Wait until you have time to complete a stage or the whole of a job. Don't pick up a piece of paper and half read it, decide it is too difficult to tackle or you haven't enough time and put it down again. You will have wasted that time deciding to put it off. And if you are in this lazy state of mind you may welcome unnecessary interruptions and compound the time-wasting further.

Top tips

The key to good time management as a leader is to:

- prioritise how you spend your time – do not allow yourself or others to waste it; control interruptions
- involve all your staff or team in improving the efficiency and effectiveness of your organisation and services you provide
- include time for thinking, doing, meeting and learning in your working day
- allow sufficient time for the unexpected throughout your working week
- delegate work whenever it is appropriate; find the right balance of delegation for important tasks such as communication – invest in your support staff so they become more confident and capable
- try only to accept delegated work without further training if you have the necessary skills, time and experience for it
- get on with essential tasks and do not procrastinate
- be assertive – learn to say 'no' often enough, to unnecessary work or taking on other people's jobs and tasks
- make effective decisions and don't look back
- put past mistakes behind you – do not ruminate over them
- review significant problems and learn to manage time better to avoid those problems in future. Review the impact of changes that you make – making realistic action plans for ways to be ever more efficient
- balance your work and leisure time in a sustainable way.

Frequently asked questions and answers

Q. *Being the leader of our nursing team takes up much more time than I anticipated when I agreed to do it. There's so much to do to ensure that the team functions well – chatting to the other nurses, listening to their problems, negotiating with the trust management etc. How can I cope with my own caseload other than step down as team leader?*
A. You could keep a log of the time it takes for the additional tasks of being team leader. I can tell you want to do the job properly and be a good and effective leader, and that takes time – that you must demonstrate to your manager. Once you have the evidence of how the time in your working week is allocated, discuss how to protect time for your leadership role with your manager, which might mean reducing your caseload.

Q. *I lead our research group and am responsible for convening our regular monthly business meetings. But we have so many items to discuss and agree that after long arguments the meetings can last up to 4 hours and people start slipping off early before we're even halfway through. Help!*
A. First review if you need to have the meetings as often as once a month. Could some of the business be dealt with by a responsible sub-committee or via chair's action? Be clear about the purpose of the meetings; and the individual items – are they for information, discussion, decision? Insist each paper gives its purpose and

guide the committee to address each appropriately (that is, no discussion on a paper that is for information only). Ask if there is any other business (AOB) at the start of the meeting so you can allow sufficient time for additional items. Ensure you have a well structured agenda, that papers are circulated in advance to allow people to read them and reflect. With good communication, freely available documents, and rapidly produced minutes, you should end up with a slicker agenda, structured discussion and timely closure.

Interactive exercise: time management is a lead issue

Which time management techniques have worked for you in the past? Which do you still do? Complete the columns in Table 9.1. Add more rows at the bottom of the Table if you use other time management techniques not included here.

Table 9.1 Checklist of approaches to time management.

Time management principles	Tried in past	Use now	Work for you
Keep time log of activities and review			
Write down tasks – prioritise them and make an action plan			
Reduce unnecessary activities			
Get work in perspective and limit time spent			
Delegate appropriately			
Go on a formal course – time for reflection			
Whenever possible handle one piece of paper once – deal with it straightaway			
Say 'No' to extra work			
Don't take on other people's jobs/tasks			
Set aside 'thinking' time			
Allow time for unexpected tasks (at least 10% of your time)			
Be brief on the phone			
Tackle one task at a time – finish it			
Prepare for meetings to be effective			
Listen carefully and so act correctly first time			
Don't procrastinate – do it now			
Do difficult tasks when you are most alert			
Other (you add your own):			

Now reflect on your own, or in discussion with a colleague or friend on the number and nature of time management techniques that you use, and those that work for you. Are there some that work for you but you rarely use? Could you do more of those that work for you more often? Could you stop doing things ostensibly to save time that do not work for you?

Chapter 10

Organisational skills

Kay Mohanna

Introduction

The benefits of good organisational skills in a leader will be enhanced performance of the workforce. We are facing many new organisational challenges in healthcare. Establishing and promoting clinical governance, involving the public and patients in meaningful ways, changing skill mix, adopting new models of working, working in truly integrated teams with alternative providers, and encouraging patients to self care, require us all to have an understanding of the current context and culture as well as a willingness to change. An effective leader will be able to steer a course around and through these challenges leading to successful implementation of service improvements

Leaders must have a clear understanding of both the formal and informal aspects of their organisation as well as all their responsibilities for strategic development and change management. Then they will be able to get the most out of the organisation and its workforce.

The formal organisation includes the hierarchy and accountability arrangements, information systems, committee structure and meetings, employment and pay issues. The informal features include relationships, the kinds of behaviours that are expected and rewarded, communication, distribution of power and how conflicts are handled.

In this chapter we will look at three aspects of an organisation that require good leadership; chairing meetings, appraisal of staff and dealing with grievances.

> The best leader is the one who has sense enough to pick the right men to do what he wants done and self-restraint enough to keep from meddling with them whilst they do it.
>
> Theodore Roosevelt

Organisational skills for leadership

Chairing meetings

When you consider organisational aspects of leadership you can recognise at least five styles:

1 **authoritarian**. Giving clear directions for specific tasks
2 **authoritative**. Stating broad objectives and delegating the detailed execution to others while accepting responsibility for the outcome

3 **democratic**. Encouraging participation to secure the benefit of the expertise of all team members
4 **task orientated**. Focusing on the task in hand and requiring a high standard of task accomplishment, regardless of other considerations
5 **developmental**. Focusing on the longer-term development of members of the team as an investment in the future.

It is when chairing meetings that someone's leadership style can best be observed. The categories are not mutually exclusive, and each style is relevant in the appropriate context as they have their own strengths. The skill of a leader is to balance their style of leadership with the desired outcomes and characteristics of team members.

Often meetings are a regular, routine part of day to day activity for responding to queries that need a quick decision, managing daily concerns or keeping channels of communication open. But from time to time you convene larger more in-depth gatherings, especially at times of change, for brainstorming new approaches to problems or when team building is required. There are however certain generic activities and behaviours that you can identify when meetings are chaired effectively:

- the purpose of the meeting should be known to all in good time before the meeting occurs
- a timetabled programme should be laid out at the planning stage – with details of aims, procedures, expected outcomes, channels or processes for feedback and review
- a good chair prepares well so that the agenda is clear and inclusive
- the exercise of getting the team together should be necessary – sufficient information should not already be available from other sources
- there should be sufficient resources allocated to the meeting – notably time
- the leader should be aware of potential conflicts of interests (e.g. competing priorities)
- involvement of all key personnel should be sought and achieved at an early stage in the process of planning the meeting
- the chair will ensure full and active participation of everyone in the meeting and that all views are heard, valued and summarised
- the meeting should consider the impacts, benefits, drawbacks of proposed changes and have enough information to be able to do so effectively
- alternative viewpoints and outcomes should be discussed, and the temptation to focus down on a solution too closely at the start should be avoided
- decisions or changes should be made as a result of the investment of time and resources in the meeting – or if they were not, the lack of changes could be justified
- the chair should ensure that meeting discussions are realistic and that explicit, timed action plans are drawn up and reviewed at a later date
- good notes must be taken and circulated to all stakeholders afterwards.

Appraisal

Identifying what motivates staff can lead to their implementation of changes that ensure more productive working. One of the best ways to discover what motivates people to perform well at work is to ask them. Some will want more money, others more time, some more flexibility in their work schedule, others to do new and more challenging tasks.

The opportunity afforded by the introduction of appraisal across the healthcare workforce is to have protected time to consider such issues. In addition you want to know if there are untapped strengths and hidden attributes that you can put to use in your organisation.

Leaders will want to get the most out of their workforce by ensuring a good fit between the work to be done and those doing it. Appraisees should be asked: 'What aspects of your current job do you enjoy and are you good at?'

Appraisal might identify any of the following as aspects that motivate a productive workforce:

- interesting and/or useful work
- a sense of achievement
- responsibility
- opportunities for career progression or professional development
- gaining new skills or competencies
- a sense of belonging to the healthcare organisation or practice or department team
- personal or written congratulations from a respected colleague or immediate superior
- public recognition
- announcement of success at team meetings
- recognising that the last job was well done and asking for an opinion of the next one
- providing specific and frequent feedback
- providing information on how the task has affected the performance of the organisation or management of a patient
- encouragement to increase their knowledge and skills to do even better
- making time to listen to ideas, complaints or difficulties
- learning from mistakes and making visible changes.

The development of a learning culture is a practical measure to enable the workforce to regularly hone their skills and knowledge and address their organisation's objectives through their delivery of high quality services. A foundation stone of the learning culture is a systematic and effective appraisal scheme that links the organisational objectives with professional and personal objectives of its staff. It provides a demonstration of a leader's commitment to the continued renewal of intellectual capital.

A good leader uses the appraisal opportunity to build relationships with their staff and identify any untapped potential as well as support them in their personal development. They use the opportunity to pool learning needs across the organisation and make appraisal relevant to the service objectives across the whole organisation.

Job satisfaction is known to protect health professionals from the effects of stress from work; so increasing job satisfaction is one of the best ways to 'stress proof' them against the pressures and demands of a busy environment. Those elements of the job that staff find stressful will be reduced if they enjoy their job, feel valued and are in control, all aspects that can be addressed through effective appraisal.

The risk of introducing appraisal to organisations the first time is that it may be perceived as performance management. Effective communication by leaders implementing this policy will be required to flag up the educational opportunity it also represents.

Dealing with grievances

All organisations have complaints, critical incidents and significant events to deal with from time to time. It is a marker of the maturity of an organisation and the skill of the leader as to how open the processes for dealing with them will be. Analysis of such incidents is one way an effective organisation can identify blind spots about organisational shortcomings and continue to develop.

Good leadership entails developing and implementing processes that aim to resolve a grievance informally at the point at which the problem arose. Many apparent concerns arise from misunderstandings that can quickly be resolved by talking the matter through. However all staff must feel that their complaints are taken seriously, are dealt with respectfully and efficiently and that the outcomes are transparent. Clearly they must be free from the worries that raising grievances might have unexpected and unwanted repercussions such as the loss of their position.

An effective staff grievance procedure:

- is easily accessible
- resolves complaints informally wherever possible
- allows speedy handling, with established time frames for action
- ensures a full and fair investigation
- respects complainants' desire for confidentiality whenever possible
- provides an effective response and appropriate redress
- feeds back into organisational systems to ensure that services are improved.

If a member of the team feels unable to bring up their problem with the person directly involved or considers that the matter has not been satisfactorily resolved, further investigation will be needed. Policies and protocols for dealing with this sort of situation should be clear and explicit, with a timescale of expected progress and the course of action to be implemented. It must be clear who is responsible for what intervention.

After full investigation leaders should ensure that the findings are shared with all parties. If a complaint is found to be malicious or vexatious then this too should be addressed and might result in disciplinary proceedings. The delicate balance of support for staff and fair investigation of all staff grievances can tax the most skilful team leader. It is much better to try and avoid such issues in the first place by effective team development initiatives and rigorous organisational structures.

Top tips

Good leadership skills in organisational matters include:

- ensuring that the organisation has a coherent commitment to quality improvement
- clear lines of accountability for quality systems

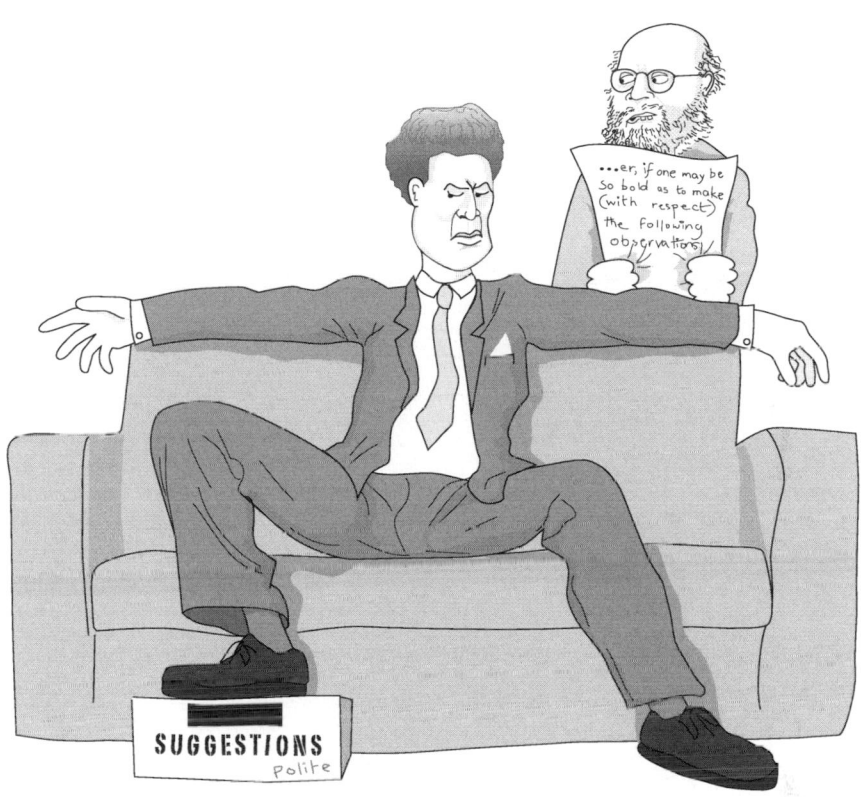

Complaint? Put it in the black hole.

- understanding the principles of equal opportunity and demonstrating best practice
- making evaluations and providing feedback on performance that is free of bias and prejudice
- effective processes for identifying and addressing poor performance
- interpreting people's rights in ways that are consistent with legislation and policies, whilst having a cultural awareness
- development and maintenance of a safe working environment for all staff identifying risks in relation to health, safety and security of employees
- supporting the development of a learning and development culture which encourages the sharing of good practice
- an open and constructive communication system including free sharing of ideas in meetings
- demonstrating good practice in processing data and information
- fostering teamwork and good working relationships throughout the organisation
- recognising and developing the leadership skills and potential of others.

Frequently asked questions and answers

Q. *We have had an anonymous complaint from an unknown member of staff against another. Are we obliged to investigate?*
A. There is no obligation, as the complaint is anonymous, but whether or not you proceed will depend to some extent on the severity of the accusation. What is the track record of the person being complained about? Has anything like this been alleged before? If the allegation is about bullying or discrimination the complainant may feel unable to put their name on the complaint for fear of reprisals. However it does make investigation and ascertainment of facts very hard. The person being complained about has a right to know the case against them. Perhaps you could appeal for the person complaining to approach you in confidence and then try to gain a mutual agreement to proceed in an open way?

Q. *A member of staff alleges that she has been passed over for promotion in favour of a colleague whom she states has less experience than her. The promoted colleague is male and she is claiming sex discrimination.*
A. Hopefully this should not be difficult to investigate and, if there are no grounds for the allegations, to defend. Annual appraisals of both members of staff should have documented their personal and professional development, the advice that has been given to them about their careers and their seniority. Under the equal opportunities legislation a case of discrimination requires a decision that disadvantaged a person because of their gender or age and cannot be justified on the basis of merit or ability. If the complainant is more qualified and able to do the job, she might have a case. If the two candidates are similarly qualified the choice may have been made on the grounds of which would fit the team better. This is not unreasonable but should be documented. What you do now is going to depend on how well your records have been kept, the person specification for the promotion opportunity and the rigor of the interview process for the new post.

Interactive exercise: analysing a stressful event

Leaders need to be aware of potential sources of 'organisational stress' at work that might affect performance, and this is an area that an effective leader will discuss with all those they appraise. It applies to you as much as to other team leaders and your team members. The exercise requires you to reflect on an area of work that has been stressful for you.

Box 10.1 Analyse a stressful event at work in relation to a leadership role.

Stage 1: write down a factual account of the stressful situation you have chosen – who was involved, the time of day, the setting and circumstances and the task/activity you or others were doing.

Stage 2: write down the reasons you perceive that caused the crisis or stressful situation.

Stage 3: write down the effects of stress on you and the other participants in the crisis or stressful situation you have chosen.

Stage 4: record how you or others might have behaved differently, or how the processes and systems in your organisation might be changed to reduce or eliminate this cause of stress from occurring again.

Discuss your analysis of the significant event with your mentor or a colleague whose perspective you value, to draw out more insights and new ideas for solutions.

Chapter 11

Dealing with problems

Veronica Wilkie and Hugh Flanagan

Introduction

Problems in performance within a healthcare setting have profound effects on patients and also on individual healthcare professionals and the systems in which they work. It has been estimated that over one-third of doctors who are the subject of a clinical negligence claim suffer from clinical depression as a result of the process.[1] The National Audit Office has estimated that £2 billion is wasted on unnecessary bed stays through errors, with a further £1 billion cost as a result of hospital acquired infections.[2] Similar findings in the United States of America estimate that more people die from medical errors than from road traffic accidents, breast cancer or AIDS taken together.[3]

Performance problems do not only affect clinical functioning, but non-clinical behaviour too. The quality of the team in the healthcare setting can have an impact on the quality of healthcare.[4] A member of a team can have all the knowledge and skills necessary for their clinical field but create problems at work through poor communication, harassment, or over or under-assertiveness. Good leadership can minimise performance problems, through an understanding of the causes of poor performance and their avoidance. And the development and support of a culture that enables the organisation to continually develop so as to be able to minimise poor performance and maximise patient safety.

> In the great majority of cases, the causes of serious failures stretch far beyond the actions of the individuals immediately involved. Safety is a dynamic, not a static situation. In a socially and technically complex field such as healthcare, a huge number of factors are at work at any one time which influence the likelihood of failure ...[5]

Dealing with problems by good leadership

Leading for an open culture

Whilst it is acknowledged that 'to err is human', organisations can minimise errors through sustaining an open and supportive culture. Historically, a culture of blame was thought to hinder the reporting and analysis of incidents which had it been otherwise might have prevented similar incidents happening again.[6] A 'no blame' culture can also create problems, as it can fail to deal with the systems and organisations that have caused an incident.[7] Far better to develop a safety culture where a team realises that mistakes and incidents happen, but can share information openly with team members and patients so that staff have fair treatment. That way there is a continual learning process in place.

Throughout healthcare, leadership is shared and happens at many levels. Clear and positive leadership with leaders that 'walk the talk' in terms of open discussion can motivate and encourage discussion throughout the team. Steps to achieve this can be done by:

- good teamwork; with effective and supporting communication
- working to maintain an open culture even in a time of rapid organisational change
- time to review policies and guidelines as a team in the light of changing evidence and circumstances
- looking at incidents in terms of why they occurred, rather than who was to blame
- supporting staff fairly when incidents happen, so that they, in turn, will support their colleagues
- acknowledging that occasionally an incident can be of a severity that demands 'suspension' from work until an assessment can be done, and having the foresight to lead and support the team members whilst this is happening
- engaging in dialogue with the wider health organisation's governance team and patient safety managers to ensure that an efficient and informed investigation is undertaken as necessary.

Barriers to reporting incidents within healthcare have been identified as a:

- professional culture that personalises failure and error, and seeks and expects perfection
- deep sense of failure for the individual
- fear of blame (enhanced by public and media attitudes)
- fear of litigation.

There are several myths to dispel when you are creating a suitable culture for dealing with problems. For instance, that if people try hard enough they will not make any errors; that if you punish people they will make fewer mistakes; and that harsh disciplinary action will lead to fewer errors.[8]

Spotting poor performance

Good leadership should enable the organisation to spot performance problems before they arise. Poor performance within a team can have a multiplicity of causes. A change in team dynamics that affects performance is discussed elsewhere (*see* Chapter 7). Other performance issues can be picked up through the running of individual and whole organisation review systems, and from monitoring by an outside agency as well as that within the organisation (e.g. the UK's clinical governance procedures for the NHS). Reasons for poor performance can be identified by looking at the issues associated with incidents (*see* Box 11.1 for example issues) and analysing what led to their occurrence.

Box 11.1 Individual and organisational markers relating to poor performance.

Individual issues
- A significant event where a patient comes to harm.
- Personality issues, e.g. outbursts of temper, harassment, low mood, poor engagement.
- Recurrent complaints by colleagues and or patients.
- Lack of knowledge demonstrated in clinical letters, referrals or in discussions, lack of knowledge within defined job descriptions for management staff.
- Activity significantly above and below the norm in a variety of parameters (patient referrals, number/type of prescriptions, treatment activity, community visits, slow procedures).
- Recurrent absences through ill health.
- Being persistently dysfunctional in team meetings.
- Refusal to engage with the team or take part in organisational meetings.

Organisational issues
- A significant event where a patient comes to harm.
- Rapid staff turnover.
- Multiple complaints from many areas within the team.
- High staff absenteeism.
- Poor communication.
- Low rate of development, with barriers put in place for staff to do continuing professional development (CPD). Little or no in-house development or CPD.
- Poor interaction with the wider organisation.
- Financial over- or under-spending.
- Activity that falls significantly above or below the norm.

Diagnosing the causes

Once a problem has been identified a good leader will put in place a way to look into the associated issues. In many cases an issue that is relatively minor can be resolved through discussion with the sharing of input from all those involved. This might be for something small and done 'on the spot', or might mean talking through the issue at a time set aside for significant event analysis, critical incident review or root cause analysis. Good chairing of this meeting should ensure that every team member's account and views are taken into consideration. Such incidents need not only be negative; good practice should also be shared, discussed and systems revised or introduced so that good practice is facilitated or sustained in the future.

Very rarely a problem or incident is so serious that significant harm may have happened or nearly happened (a 'near miss'). In the UK the National Patient Safety Agency has developed an incident decision tree to help organisations deal with such issues.[9]

Looking at the incident in a structured way to 'dissect' all possible causes is sometimes called a 'root cause analysis'. The stages of such an analysis are illustrated in Figure 11.1.

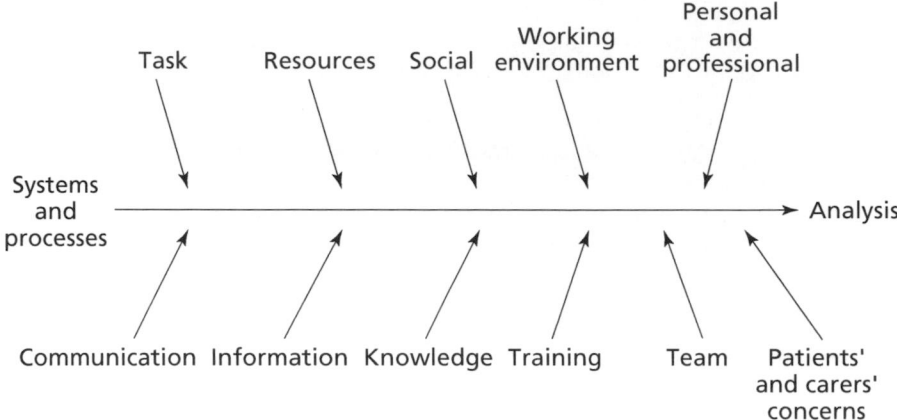

Figure 11.1 Issues to consider when analysing a problem (adapted from *Seven Steps to Patient Safety for Primary Care*).[9]

Following the analysis it is vital that members of the team or the investigators reflect on what has happened and develop recommendations. The team leader should define each individual's responsibility for implementing the recommendations and have a very clear idea of the timescale. Without this aspect of leadership, the time and energy spent in looking at the performance issues may be lost. Many healthcare organisations have, or are developing, policies to share learning from significant events. In this respect, healthcare organisations are taking the lead from other industries to establish clear and accountable reporting processes so that the whole organisation can benefit.[10]

Top tips

- Sustaining leadership when there are problems requires you to have a multiplicity of skills – so consider and address your development needs.
- Developing an open and supportive culture can help an organisation to learn and develop systems so that future mistakes are minimised.
- Look to learn what led an individual to behave in the way that triggered a problem, rather than necessarily apportion blame.
- Remember that a serious incident will be traumatic for the patient, family and healthcare professional involved.
- Punishing individuals without having a clear sense of the whole issue will lead to non-reporting of future problems and continuance of unsafe practice.
- Spotting performance issues involves having an understanding of the functioning of the healthcare organisation from a variety of sources of information from within and without the organisation.
- Diagnosing what leads to the performance issue(s) requires the whole system to be examined in a mutually supportive and systematic fashion, without collusion or superficial 'fixes'.
- Remember that an individual's behaviour at work is determined by conditions and events in their workplace as well as their home circumstances.

- Always put in place a plan for following up the extent to which recommendations have been implemented.
- It is common for there to be an underlying health problem when someone is underperforming – so involve occupational health earlier rather than later in your clarification of the concerns.

Frequently asked questions and answers

Q. *What sort of problems lead to performance issues by a healthcare professional?*
A. Increasingly, research in this field has shown that in many cases performance is affected by more than one issue. It is uncommon for a healthcare professional to perform poorly because of lack of knowledge alone. There are very often issues concerning their personality, their working environment and their health which lead to a lack of knowledge or clinical skills. The team in turn may also suffer and a downward spiral start for more than one individual. A lack of leadership in the organisation can exacerbate poor performance by individuals.[11]

Q. *What should I do if I suspect that one of my colleagues has a health problem?*
A. Health issues are commonly found in people with performance issues. The healthcare and pharmaceutical industries have experienced unparalleled increases in the reporting of stress by their staff. In the NHS 40% of workers say that they work under stress, 74% state that stress has contributed to ill health and one third report ill health.[12] Working in a healthcare environment may make individuals reluctant to seek help. As with any issue of concern, discussing your fears with the individual may encourage them to seek help, if they are working in a supportive culture. A review of their role at work may be needed. If you feel that they have a mental or physical health issue that is putting patients at risk, and you are unable to engage with the individual you should discuss your concerns with a senior manager or clinician (or the clinical governance lead in your trust).

Q. *Where should I go for advice on performance procedures?*
A. Your organisation should have a procedure for dealing with issues of performance. In-house procedures should reflect those of the overarching organisation that are responsible to them (the NHS Clinical Governance Support Team and National Patient Safety Agency may advise – by phone or from their websites and tools).[13,14] The various professional regulatory bodies have clear guidance on what to do if performance problems are apparent and what next steps to take.

Q. *How can I as a leader get support when dealing with stressful issues?*
A. You should hopefully have someone within your team to go to for support (if not there is a big team issue!). It will also be useful to speak to another trusted colleague or your mentor who may have had similar experiences, as well as those who are in a position professionally to support you. You need to harvest all those resources that have been put in place to help you to succeed, when leading in times of stress.

Q. *Are there procedures or resources to help rehabilitate people with serious performance issues?*
A. Most healthcare systems will have supportive and systematic processes for rehabilitation. Where serious performance problems occur, an external review

body will often give very specific advice on retraining and re-assessment. The details will vary according to the profession and the country. Details can be obtained from the regulatory body. There are a very few cases where their problem is thought to be sufficiently severe to prevent the individual working again within their professional field.

Interactive exercise: get on the case when you are dealing with problems

As an individual, reflect on the case below using Figure 11.1 to explore the range of potential causes of the performance problem described below. Then, or alternatively, discuss the case in a small group, maybe with others in your team at work. Using a theoretical exercise such as this case review can help your team to discuss group rules and terms of reference before you repeat the exercise based on a problem issue in your organisation. You could change the roles in the case to try and reflect a similar scenario to that which has happened or could happen in your workplace.

The scenario: you have a senior role in your healthcare organisation. As you are about to leave one of the nurses asks if she can have a quick word with you. She describes one of her nurse colleagues as becoming very difficult to deal with. She frequently shouts at the other team members, is often late, and rarely follows up on clinical issues. The nurse is concerned that other team members are having to check patients' notes to ensure that they have been appropriately dealt with. She describes an incident when they tried to alert this nurse about a very poorly looking man who was waiting to see her. She was abusive and refused to see him as 'she had other patients waiting too ...' The patient had to be sent to A&E.

You go to see this member of staff the next day. She appears flustered and hassled. She attributes most of her problems to the pressure of work and the patient targets which she feels are unrealistic. 'On top of this, I have a divorce to contend with and I'm unable to drive and have to deal with the vagaries of public transport.'

Speculate on the potential causes of this problem case using the categories in Figure 11.1. Reflect on your own particular issue and analyse the problem; or discuss the fictional case with a colleague. Then think of some strategies you could use for sorting it out.

References

1 Donaldson L. *Making Amends*. A consultation paper setting out proposals for reforming the approach to clinical negligence in the NHS. A Report by the Chief Medical Officer. London: Department of Health; 2003. www.dh.gov.uk/assetRoot/04/06/09/45/04060945.pdf.

2 National Audit Office. *A Safer Place for Patients. Learning to Improve Patient Safety*. London: National Audit Office; 2005.

3 Institute of Medicine (IOM). *To Err is Human: building a safer health system*. Washington DC: National Academy Press; 2000.

4 National Clinical Assessment Authority. *Teamwork and Performance, in Understanding Performance Difficulties in Doctors*. Section 8. London: NCAA; 2004.

5   Department of Health. *An Organisation with a Memory*. Report of an expert group on learning from adverse events in the NHS. London: Department of Health; 2000.

6   Royal College of Nursing. *Clinical Governance: how nurses can get involved*. London: Royal College of Nursing; 2000.

7   National Clinical Assessment Service. *Back on Track. Restoring Doctors and Dentists to Safe Professional Practice.* Consultation and Framework Document. London: Department of Health; 2005.

8   Leap LL. Striving for perfection. *Clin Chem.* 2002; **48**(11): 1871–2.

9   National Patient Safety Agency. Step 6: learn and share safety lessons. In: *Seven Steps to Patient Safety for Primary Care.* London: NPSA; 2006.

10 Department of Health and Chief Medical Officer. Chapter 3 Learning to Fly. In: *On the State of Public Health: annual report of the Chief Medical Officer 2005.* DH; 2006. www.dh.gov.uk/assetRoot/04/13/73/70/04137370.pdf.

11 Pendleton D, King J. Values and Leadership. *BMJ.* 2002; **325**: 1352–5.

12 Spurgeon P. Managing Stress in Healthcare Organisations. In: Spurgeon P, editor. *The New Face of the NHS.* London: Royal Society of Medicine Press Ltd; 1998.

13 www.cgsupport.nhs.uk

14 www.npsa.nhs.uk

Chapter 12

Being a leader through times of change

Bev Norton

Introduction

Within any organisation there will inevitably be change. Any change, no matter how small and seemingly insignificant it may appear to you, will have an impact on others within the organisation. So it is important to recognise and predict where this change will improve the working of the organisation and where there may be an adverse effect that you should address.

At the highest level change may be imposed through national initiatives, directives or new legislation. These may require organisations to behave differently, such as from the introduction of disability discrimination, changes in taxation, or safety standards.

It may be that the organisation wants to bring about change, such as relocating to alternative premises, introducing different working hours for staff, or modifying clinical procedures.

Some types of change directly affect individuals at work, such as when working with new colleagues or clients. Sometimes changed personal circumstances at home impact on the person's behaviour or attitudes at work.

As a leader how you deal with change will vary according to the type or degree of change, the commitment to the change by individual(s) or organisation(s) affected and people's levels of engagement within the process.

> Everyone thinks of changing the world but nobody thinks of changing themselves.
>
> Leo Tolstoy

Leadership through change

Change seems to be constant in the NHS and that is one of the biggest challenges a leader faces. Any change, no matter how large or small, impacts on the individuals within an organisation. They in turn impact on other colleagues and associated stakeholders and the productivity and development of the organisation itself. As a leader you will be supporting individuals through the change process to deliver the set outcome or other appropriate outcome(s).

The starting point to any change process is to recognise what the type of change is, whether or not the need for change is imposed by an external source, is due to development or is an innovative idea from within the team. Change that is imposed will produce negative feelings in those it concerns compared with the

type of change where the person has been invited to contribute or has partici-
pated. Thus a successful leader will try to ensure that consultation takes place to
discuss and develop a strategy for undertaking the change even when faced with
a 'must do' requirement to make the change.

The amount of control that a person has over the change will determine their
commitment to the new organisation or process. How they react will also relate
to their previous experience, their present level of security as well as their own
individual personality. We all have a comfort zone which allows us to work
within defined and familiar boundaries. Going beyond these may invoke fear of
the unknown and unfamiliar challenges. Different individuals will see change as
giving them an opportunity to push out the boundaries and enjoy the experience,
whilst others will be fearful and hold back from the perceived 'danger' zone.

How people adapt to change will be determined by the way that the change is
introduced and the responsiveness of the person(s) facing the change. If a person
lacks the will to engage, they may adopt disruptive behaviour, become cynical
and possibly resign from their post.

Figure 12.1 is based on a bereavement/counselling model. It illustrates the
emotions that a person may experience when in a situation of change and a
common ensuing cycle of behaviour.

Just like the estate agent who relies on good location – a leader of change relies
on communication, communication and even better communication! But communication is not just telling team members about a change. The leader needs to
actively discuss with and listen to affected members, provide information and
receive feedback. Throughout the process the leader needs to be aware of, and
understand, the uncertainty and anxiety of those affected by the change. They
should address these feelings through appropriate forums and shared processes,

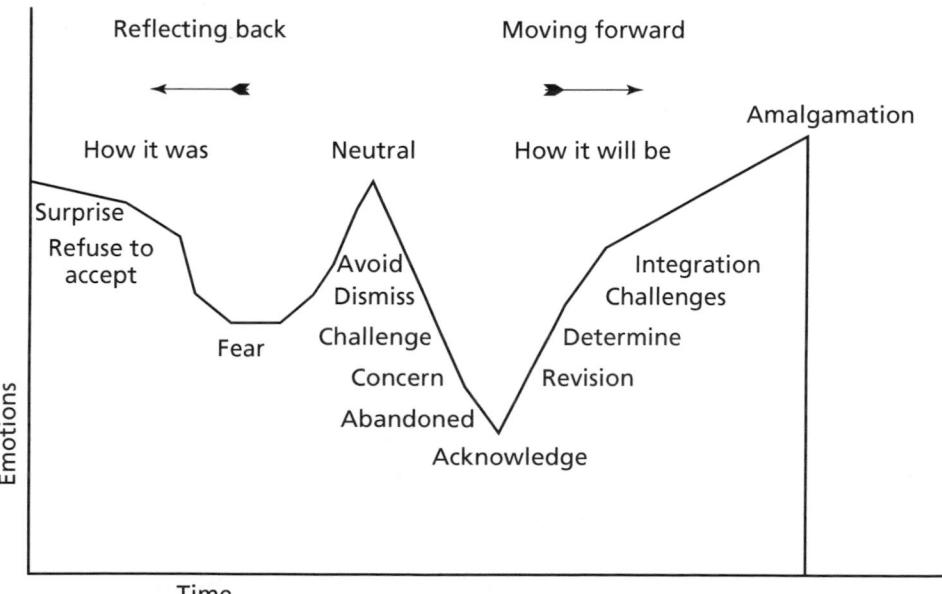

Figure 12.1 Illustration of possible emotional and behavioural responses to change.

rather than dismiss these emotions as irrelevant. Due to an individual's own personal emotional state and biases, they will put their own construction on various pieces of information and alter the meaning to suit their own preferences and zone of understanding. Leaders need to overcome the way that different individuals modify the information given out by delivering important messages through a series of media, which might include visual presentations, discussions and clear written notes to reinforce key messages.

An ability to motivate others is a core skill required in a leader. How individuals are informed of an impending change will affect their attitude towards accepting it and their performance during the change process. To achieve maximum commitment teams should work together under strong leadership on developing the change process and achieving commitment. Any organisational change will require behavioural change on the part of the individuals concerned, not just at a superficial level when the 'boss is looking,' but internalised into new processes.

It may be necessary for individuals to develop new skills for an organisation to undertake the change. Thus within the process of developing the change, time and resources should be set aside for the education and development of team members. Identifying people's learning needs will provide further opportunities for them to expand their personal portfolios and succeed in a new situation. An organisational change affects the equilibrium within a team which typically moves through a cycle of four stages as members progress together: storming, reforming, norming to performing (*see* page 48). The maturity of the organisation will impact upon the time that team members spend in each phase.

Top tips

- Be clear about what you are trying to change and the reasons for that change.
- Determine if there is only one acceptable outcome or if you can work towards different solutions.
- Recognise how the change will impact on individuals and the organisation. Are team members used to change and flexible in their approach or is the culture within the organisation one of a 'steady state'?
- Understand the pace of change that is required. Is it a legislative requirement and thus imposed? Must it be achieved within a deadline? Is it essential and required within a limited timescale? Or is it desirable and there is time for full involvement, commitment and development of those affected?
- As a leader of change remember that it will also impact on you. Be prepared to plan how you yourself will move through the process and predetermine your own fears and opportunities for development as part of the change.
- Within any situation of change recognise the limitations – these may be self imposed, real or imagined.
- Throughout any change a leader will be supporting and motivating others. Consider how members of your team feel about change, whether they are keen to embrace change or reluctant to do so. Understand the importance of motivation and how it should be matched to the needs and feelings of your team members as far as possible.
- Always check that you have communicated effectively with everyone else, via an appropriate media; and confirmed that the communications have been understood.

- Learn from change. Even the smallest change can provide lessons for you as the leader on how you and others have reacted to the situation.
- Never underestimate the time and effort that change takes. Remember the possibility of storming and conflict, and the need for a period of reforming before the organisation can be re-established under a state of normality.
- The performance of the organisation has to continue even through prolonged periods of change. This will take energy, understanding and support of staff.
- Implementing change successfully requires planning, engagement, agility and commitment. As a leader you need to demonstrate that flexibility yourself, and your own motivational and facilitation skills.

Frequently asked questions and answers

Q. *How do I as a leader manage the morale and motivation in my organisation during a change?*
A. To manage change requires that you have good managerial skills of influencing, coaching and motivating. As a leader you should recognise how individuals will react to the introduction of change. Consider how people will be influenced by their peer groups and ensure that you can motivate them to be 'on side'. Motivation can be through a reward of a financial nature or related to their professional development or values. It is important to establish what others are seeking, to be able to reward their acceptance of the change to move on from the status quo.

Q. *How can I lead a change that I don't believe in?*
A. This is probably the hardest challenge. Recognise the requirement for change and that potentially being disadvantaged by the change as an individual is not an uncommon occurrence in the health service. In this instance you as the leader have to rise above your own personal prejudices and create an atmosphere of calm and development. Attempt to put forward the advantages to be gained for the organisation and many of the individuals within it, from the change. The disaffected leader needs to rationalise the proposals and ensure that the outcomes and goals are clearly identified, focusing on the positive and being strong enough to avoid unwarranted criticism. As a leader your role is to undertake the task and for some the endpoint of the change cannot always be perfect.

Q. *How do I deal with negative, disruptive responses associated with a change?*
A. There may be a variety of reactions to a situation of change, the strength of which are proportional to the impact of the change on individuals. Some team members will retreat into a shell and clam up. You will have to encourage them to open up and express their concerns. Others may display disruptive behaviour such as anger and cynicism. Then you should provide them with the space and opportunity to express these negative feelings and as much support and opportunity for rational debate and flexibility in the development of a strategy for undertaking the change as is feasible.

Interactive exercise: all change – look to it

Identify a change that you have undertaken or been involved with, in an organisation – your practice or trust.

Draw a time line of how you approached the process of change and plot on it where the following actions took place and the impact of each. The list below may help with key tasks and words.

1 Identification of change required:
   - who made the decision to change?
   - who was involved in agreeing the planned outcome(s)?
   - was the initial anticipated outcome the change that actually took place?
   - if not, when and how was the change made?
2 Were the goals set out clearly?
3 How was the process communicated to others?
   - What channels of communication were used?
   - How many people were involved?
   - What was their reaction to the proposals for change?
   - Were there opportunities to change the planned outcome(s)?
4 Did you have to deal with people's:
   - positive reactions?
   - negative reactions?
5 How did these reactions change over time?
6 What influenced the change in your own or other people's attitudes?
7 Did morale drop during the process? If so, what was it that you or others did that re-established morale within the organisation?
8 Was an analysis undertaken after the change had happened to ascertain the effectiveness of the change(s) made? Did that include gathering information that allowed you to deduce why the planned change(s) was effective or failed to work out in real life?

Chapter 13

Leading research

Ruth Chambers

Introduction

As a research lead you have a whole range of roles to play. You will be the role model for your team, being ultimately responsible for the standards of research practised. If you are an experienced leader, researchers in your team will be to some extent your apprentices, especially if they are at early stages in their research careers. Your team may be dependent on you for their livelihoods, and the extent of research funding. You will encourage them, chivvy them on to meet deadlines, challenge them to achieve their best and be their critical friend as to their research outputs.

You might be a mentor to a researcher just starting out in their career or midway through and needing some help in progressing. If so, you might advise them about research opportunities locally, or further afield, even abroad. You might discuss various niche fields where it will be easier for them to make their name and raise their profile. You could introduce them to research networks of experienced researchers with whom they might collaborate in future.

> The one quality particular to human beings is the need to know 'why' and those in leadership positions who forget this will not remain leaders for very long.
>
> Neil Goodwin, Chief Executive,
> Greater Manchester Strategic Health Authority
> HSJ columnist, 2006

Being a good research leader

Box 13.1 summarises the behaviour of good leadership in an academic environment.

> **Box 13.1** Good university leadership from the perspective of 20 academic leaders.[1]
>
> - Being innovative and orientated towards change.
> - Wanting one's department to be a major force.
> - Knowing when and how to compromise, and how to accommodate dissenters.
> - Asking what you are trying to do, and why your methods for doing it may not be as successful as they should be.

- Focusing on students.
- Questioning 'sacred cows'.
- Doing things differently.
- Giving people freedom so that new ideas can surface.
- Being able to change your leadership style when necessary.
- Being an example to your colleagues.
- Being a person who networks and knows what's going on.
- Relating to people in a congenial way.
- Understanding where people are coming from.
- Getting feedback from your constituents.
- Knowing the boundaries of what you can achieve.

Multiskilled in the research process and training others. As a research team leader you will require skills for every part of the research process, even though you will delegate components of the research programme to researchers, project managers and administrative staff in your teams. A research team is usually fairly compact, with members being prepared to be flexible and able to adapt to take on various tasks and roles as the need arises. You will be training others in the team so that you can gradually delegate more and more of the work of the research project as they become more competent and confident. As leader you will be selecting the skill mix of your research teams and be the driving force in establishing good teamworking.

Lead responsibility for resources. You will ensure that funding gained is spent according to the agreed budget or justify why not. Anticipating the resources needed is an art. You need to predict the funding required to complete the research project in line with the research protocol so that sufficient fieldwork or data collection is undertaken to address the research hypothesis with findings that have the power to answer the research question(s). You'll seek new funding to sustain the research team and skills base you are building up to enhance your track record in research specialty fields. You will keep a tight rein on resources so that you can cover any shortfalls in creative ways – for instance if a skilled member of the research team leaves their post midway through the project or takes sickness absence or goes off on maternity leave; or you need to replace equipment unexpectedly. Your team will expect you to preserve enough funding to support their attendance at training activities or conferences where they can present their work and network with other researchers – an integral part of a researcher's professional life.

Good employer practices. Hopefully your human resources department will aid you in appointing staff and their employment in general. But as the research project lead you should know about equity and diversity, providing equal opportunities for your staff, supporting their personal and professional development, undertaking appraisal and personal review, providing fair references, and establishing a work environment that enables them to work effectively.

Inspiring your team. As the leader you'll want to inspire your team members so that they are committed to achieving your research goals and the values that you are striving for. A really key research question with potential to do good will help to inspire those working with you. You may be focused on organisational goals to evolve a high profile research department which specialises in new research fields or with niche areas. Or you may present more specific goals to your team that are relevant to the individual research projects upon which they are employed. Individual team members will have personal goals too – to develop skills in various strands of research methodology, to attend national and international conferences and undertake other activities that enhance their CVs and networks.

Communicating your research results. The essential element in undertaking research is letting others know about your findings, whether they are positive or negative. So as a leader you will strive to disseminate news about your method and results in research papers that are good enough to be published in internationally acclaimed peer reviewed journals. Seminars, workshops and conference presentations are the way that the research community share research findings, discuss results and challenge others' work. Books and articles may develop the research findings further, setting the research in context or applying it in creative ways. As a leader you will encourage your team to learn these communication and dissemination skills, so that they gradually can become the lead for the writing of the papers or presenting the results, or planning and delivering workshops.

Probity. Ethical practice is at the centre of any research. That means submitting a research ethics application and abiding by the agreed protocol unless the ethics committee agrees otherwise for justifiable reasons as the project progresses. It means not double funding a research programme without the various sponsors' knowledge and agreement that they are paying for the same work. It means ensuring that any other underpinning research is referenced and that no one else's work is plagiarised. In all this, the leader should be scrupulously honest and transparent; a role model of probity for all team members and being alert to any malpractice in others.

Top tips

- Stay focused on your own specialty field and build your profile around that.
- Be open to other people's ideas in formulating your research questions so that you don't get stale.
- Consider how to maintain your research programme so that it is of interest and regarded as topical by potential sponsors.
- Don't let your experience and expertise dominate your research team to the extent that team members doubt the worth of their contribution and become passive members.
- As leader you have to deliver your research project – so you need to ensure that there are completer-finishers in your team if you are not to end up doing the majority of the work yourself or with unfinished projects.
- Choose your research team so that they have a good mix of experience and attributes.
- Encourage delegation in your research teams – providing the necessary support and training for team members to take on new tasks and responsibilities.
- Keep a regular check of your planned timelines for your research projects and take action if progress is poor in any component of your intended programmes.

- Continually assess the extent of risk that any stage of your research project will not happen (e.g. poor recruitment of subjects); and introduce new activities that minimise those risks (e.g. generating good communication to people in positions to recruit subjects on your behalf).
- Take every opportunity to present your research work, giving credit to team members who have contributed and acknowledging sponsors and supporters.
- Involve anyone relevant to shaping and undertaking your research at all stages, such as patients or members of the public, your team members – listening to and valuing their opinions, and responding appropriately in developing your projects or research programmes.
- Be a good role model as to ethical practice throughout the research process, from competing for funds, to designing your research protocols, undertaking research to agreed processes and interpreting the results, acknowledging others' work, and disseminating results in a fair and balanced way.

Frequently asked questions and answers

Q. *Do you think a strong research leader should focus their research programme on their own organisation? Surely if you start working closely or collaborating with other research departments or organisations as research funders often propose, you are risking someone from outside trying to take over as leader and triggering in-fighting, and that cannot be good in the long run.*

A. These days it is rare to do research alone or in isolation from other research departments. You need to collaborate with other researchers and other organisations to bring in their diversity and experience to solve a research question from various perspectives or with a range of skills you could not usually expect to find in a single organisation. Sponsors look for wide-based research groupings where their range of experience and diverse characteristics give a strong base to the research programme that is commissioned, and increase the likelihood of the research being worthwhile and adding to the international evidence base. So it is up to you as a research leader to negotiate individual research programmes within a research portfolio or to agree clear responsibilities and accountability arrangements so that no individual leaders feel threatened or undermined.

Q. *As a research leader how do I ensure that I and my team get the recognition we deserve for our research achievements and protect our work from being exploited by others, including the research sponsors or our employers?*

A. If the research is concerned with inventing a new way of doing something – in a practical or technical sense, then you as the leader will need to be familiar with copyright, patenting and intellectual property right procedures to preserve your work and research outputs. Your personal rights as opposed to those of the research sponsor should have been specified in your research contract before work started, so that there is no dispute or misunderstanding. Your employer may have included information about your rights in the terms and conditions of your individual employment contracts – have a look and try to re-negotiate your position if you do not consider it fair.

Interactive exercise: undertake a significant event analysis of a problem relating to your research leadership

Your aim will be to reduce or change the nature of any 'hazard' or reduce the frequency/extent of any problem issue. If prevention is impossible, you could alter the ways in which you respond to the issue, or improve your ability to recognise and deal with related problems. Work through the following nine stages.

Stage 1: describe a problem situation – who was involved, what time of day, what task or activity were you or others doing. The situation should be a frequent problem (e.g. stages in a research project taking longer than predicted), an important problem with significant effects (e.g. overspending of research budget), or an infrequent event that when it occurs has far-reaching effects (e.g. a skilled researcher leaving midway through the project), costly in terms of time or resources. It must be a problem or issue which you can reasonably expect to be able to reduce or control or eliminate (e.g. for the examples given here – by better time management, better financial control system, succession planning).

Stage 2: set a sensible target to aim at in reducing, controlling or eliminating the problem that you hope to achieve after you have introduced a new system to tackle it.

Stage 3: plan to address the significant problem, describing the expected outcomes, anticipated benefits and disadvantages. Discuss your proposal with everyone involved at work. Obtain the agreement of anyone who may be concerned by your proposed changes. Amend your plans in the light of others' comments.

Stage 4: prepare to carry out your plan – obtaining or buying any equipment, training yourself or others if new skills are required, making other resource or organisational arrangements.

Stage 5: record your current performance as a baseline before making any changes.

Stage 6: introduce and carry out the intervention (for example your new system or using new equipment, training team members to be able to substitute or succeed others). Record new performance measures.

Stage 7: compare your new performance with your old performance, and with your initial target. Has your target been reached?

Stage 8: feed back information about the comparison of performance (i.e. Stage 7 results), outcomes of intervention(s) and the improvements or changes to those involved in, or affected by, your initiative. Discuss as a work team and agree further changes if your target is still not met.

Stage 9: monitor performance 3–6 months later; that is review how you are doing in addressing the problem you have focused on, compared to where you were when you started out (at Stage 1). Reinforce any interventions and/or changes etc. you have introduced as necessary to sustain your improvements.

Reference

1   Ramsden P. *Learning to Lead in Higher Education*. London: Routledge; 1998.

Chapter 14

Is it management or leadership?

Peter Spurgeon and Robert Cragg

Introduction

The current focus upon the importance of leadership has served to undermine the value and contribution of management. At its most polarised the debate about leadership and management has tended to see leadership as 'good' and management as 'bad'. This plays to the argument that people do not want to be managed, seeing it as bureaucratic and controlling; but are happy to follow the heroic leader towards a vision (sometime a little hazy) of a better future.

The essence of the debate is that leaders have a concern with the future and with people in the system, whilst managers are focused upon greater efficiency within the here and now. Inevitably the relationship between the two concepts management and leadership is more complex than this with any distinction between the two being somewhat blurred at the edges.

The importance of the issue and why it may be helpful to be clear as to what we mean by the terms *manager* and *leader* is in part to do with how we train and develop people to gain the appropriate skills. But perhaps more critically, how we recognise what types of skills and approaches people need to apply to a particular task.

> Management is efficiency in climbing the ladder of success. Leadership determines whether the ladder is leaning against the right wall.
>
> Covey[1]

Distinguishing between management and leadership

Much of this book has been concerned with how individuals display leadership in terms of their types of behaviours, and in a range of circumstances. Where does the process of management fit within these different situations? Is it a slightly more mundane and constrained process largely sidelined when the more powerful force of leadership comes into play? Or is it an integral component of leadership? Or the building blocks upon which leadership can develop?

A classic, possibly stereotypical view is of the manager as being primarily administrative, working to a short-term viewpoint, within the current systems and structures. The focus is upon making that which exists as efficient as possible. In contrast, the leader takes a longer-term perspective and seeks to initiate change for the better, to interest and inspire people to commit to a vision of what the organisation could be like.

An understanding of the context goes some way to resolving this apparent dichotomy between management and leadership. The basic functions of management – planning, budgeting, organising, controlling resources and problem solving are vital for the smooth running of any organisation; without them anarchy may result. These managerial activities though are most appropriate when organisations and the society around them are stable and relatively predictable. The constant and continual change occurring in society and the NHS in particular goes some way to explain why such a premium is placed upon leadership. If organisations need to adapt and change to new circumstances then leaders who challenge, motivate and inspire others towards a new vision are critical. The link between government demand for change in the NHS and their advocacy of the need for better leadership in all healthcare settings, is clear.

But thinking of management and leadership in this way can result in assigning people to roles labelled *manager* or *leader*. It implies too that individuals are captured in these roles and that they cannot move between them. This is clearly absurd. Managers often have responsibility for change and major implementation programmes where they will need to communicate and convince other staff of the merits of pursuing altered goals and tasks. This will feel like a leadership function; though of course it may be that some individual managers are poor at fulfilling this particular aspect of their role. This then for that individual might become a dividing point between their capacity as a manager and their inability to perform as a leader.

Does it work the other way round? Can an individual operate as a leader without being a capable manager? The answer has to be yes in terms of the charismatic leader who can articulate an inspirational vision of the future but has little notion of how to operationalise the necessary steps in getting there.

The focus of leadership as involving personal relationships is reinforced by Checkland[2] who when writing about 'soft' systems thinking emphasised the need to maintain relationships, as opposed to 'hard' systems thinking, with its emphasis on goal seeking behaviour.

Delivering and maintaining change inspired by leaders, requires management expertise. Thus the two functions support and complement one another. They vary in emphasis and are more or less appropriate at different times depending on circumstances. Both roles are needed but it is clear that some managers will be able to offer leadership in addition, whilst some cannot. Equally many outstanding leaders are also very competent managers – but that is not necessarily the case for all leaders.

> Allman states that:
>
> It is possible to have too much or too little of either. Strong management with no leadership tends to entrench an organisation in deadly bureaucracy. Strong leadership with no management risks chaos, and the organisation itself may be threatened as a result.[3]

Top tips

1 Management is most appropriate when:
   - the focus of the management process has an impact on the way that the current situation is defined

- the way that the task is structured is constrained and there are limited available options
- the task is limited to a specific and limited area of work with clear boundaries
- the work being undertaken is well understood and exists within an existing set of parameters
- the environment in which the task is conducted is stable and predictable
- the most important outcome of the task is improved efficiency.

2 Leadership is most appropriate when:
- ability goes beyond what is currently being done and involves developing a longer term vision
- the task is not routine and requires innovative thinking 'outside the box'
- there is a need to inspire and motivate others in undertaking the task
- there is a need to establish momentum and keep things moving in a new direction in order to be successful
- the task is required because the external environment is unstable and changing rapidly
- the focus of the task is upon engaging people, not doing a task.[4]

Frequently asked questions and answers

Q. *I have just joined a new general practice. I was bowled over by the practice team when I first met them whilst looking round the practice before I decided to apply for a GP partnership with them. Their ideas and enthusiasm seemed second to none. But a few months on we still seem to be finding it difficult to turn many of our ideas into reality. It isn't just me that feels like this – some of my GP partners have commented too about how we're all talk and not much action. What can we do?*

A. It is apparent that you have joined a group of innovators and leaders. Their inclination is to work in isolation, doing their very best for patients. They are most likely providing excellent care. However it seems that they are not interested in the system, how it operates or what they need to do for the good of the practice organisation overall. This group of 'leaders' will be facilitated in achieving their goals by a much stronger management process. You should recommend either the appointment of a first class practice manager or that the existing manager should go on a development course so that a more effective managerial infrastructure can be developed. Another option might be to recruit a deputy practice manager who can focus on establishing new systems. Or the GPs might each take on selected management functions.

Q. *Under the NHS reforms a new practice with links to the private sector has opened relatively near to our practice and seems to be attracting patients. What should our solid, competent practice do in response?*

A. Your analysis seems to suggest that you will need to create significant changes in the way your practice operates. This will be a major leadership challenge as many of the staff have probably been there for some time and are likely to believe that the new way of doing things will fizzle out once the newness has worn off. If you take on the leadership role, you will need to develop a clear vision of what the practice could be like, the changes needed and how you can inspire your colleagues. Your leadership should enable staff to accept the values inherent in this new approach as well as what they will need to do to make it happen. You will need to demonstrate high level leadership skills throughout the transition.

Interactive exercise: getting the balance right

Consider specific members of the team or general practice in which you work, for example, certain individuals amongst your GP or practice nurse colleagues or the practice manager. Think about their typical contributions to meetings and discussions and consider whether they exhibit primarily managerial or leadership behaviours. Reflect on the balance of the managerial and leadership make-up of the team and how the skill mix might be improved so that the team is more productive and works more effectively.

Identify an organisational problem or issue that is current or has happened recently. Analyse the demands of the task or problem in terms of whether it required more or less managerial or leadership skills. Reflect upon whether you and your team are offering the appropriate balance of management and leadership skills for a successful outcome. Discuss your thinking with another colleague. Make a plan for managerial and leadership development for team members as appropriate to the issue you have considered or you anticipate in other forthcoming tasks.

References

1   Covey SR. *The Habits of Highly Effective People*. Philadelphia: Running Press; 1989.
2   Checkland P. From optimising to learning: a development of systems thinking for the 1990s. *J Occup Research Soc.* 1985; **36**(9): 757–67.
3   Allman S. *Leadership Strategies that Work.* 2003. http://allmanconsulting.com/books.html.
4   Gardener JW. *On Leadership*. New York: The Free Press; 1990.

Chapter 15

Leading amongst equals

Peter Spurgeon and Robert Cragg

Introduction

Whatever our particular role or form of employment most of us find ourselves working in different settings within and across our working lives. We may come together with new and changing groups of people on a quite frequent basis, perhaps in various project teams. Equally, others may be part of a relatively stable group that meets regularly but infrequently to deal with critical common issues or special interest areas.

Some form of leadership function will be in operation during these gatherings – of equals. In some circumstances this may be quite formal and the leader role is designated and clear cut. Increasingly though this is not the case with more informal, loosely structured groupings forming for a purpose. Moreover, the individuals in such groups may well be peers or at least similar in terms of status and contributions. In these circumstances the location of the leadership role is less obvious. Should it be by the election and therefore consensus of others – a very formal process for an informal group? Or will it just emerge and perhaps crucially change, over the lifetime of the group?

This chapter addresses the issue of how leadership operates when you are working with peers or equals and what might be the most effective approach you could take when you are leading in such a situation.

> A complex adaptive system is a collection of individual agents with freedom to act in ways that are not always totally predictable, and whose actions are interconnected so that one agent's actions change the context for other agents.
>
> Plsek and Greenhalgh 2001[1]

Making leadership work amongst equals

The early ideas about leadership and the dominant concept for most of the last century has been to view leadership as a very individual characteristic. Attempts have been made to determine what it is that makes one person stand out from others, and therefore become the leader. Researchers have searched for 'enduring personal characteristics – that distinguish leaders from followers, and 'effective' from 'ineffective' leaders'.[2] The whole approach known as the trait theory (*see* page 33 too) emphasised the notion of charisma exercised by one 'special' individual who whatever the situation was likely to emerge as the leader because they had a set of particular characteristics. The focus on the charismatic leader was a product of its time as part of a society with a limited number of well-educated individuals and an elitist hierarchical structure.

The search though was largely futile on two grounds. Firstly, by definition, the special charisma sought whilst existing in a few people was likely to be rare and therefore unhelpful in developing leadership. Secondly, the characteristics that did emerge as describing charisma – such as self confidence, energy levels, dominance – were not in themselves defining and could well be found in others in a variety of different situations who were not necessarily leaders.

The relative failure of the approach described above does though offer insights and new ways of providing leadership in the social context of today. There are three critical strands that have changed how we need to operate:

1 The emphasis upon teamwork. This means that most people will function in multidisciplinary teams of peers where the role of the leader is negotiable and may alternate between people, depending on the team's issues and circumstances.
2 An expanded educated population with their own expectations and a desire to influence things for themselves. Traditional hierarchies and high status groups have been replaced in some instances by individuals with a legitimate desire to be involved in the decision making process in their organisation or more generally.
3 The complexity of modern society. The nature of issues to be tackled require people with a range of problem solving skills, unlikely to be found in a single person.

Inevitably then leadership itself will need to be a more complex process to cope with these challenges. An early appreciation of this came in the distinction made by many between a 'hard' and 'soft' leadership model, or task-centred versus person-centred approach. The task-oriented leader is typically concerned with the immediate task in hand and achieving the goals or outcomes required. In urgent or time restricted contexts this rather directive style may be absolutely appropriate. However it is difficult for a task leader who strives, pushes and drives towards achievement to undertake the softer more social, harmonising form of leadership aimed at bringing everyone in the group along the same route, retaining and sustaining their commitment and belief.[3] The two functions are often incompatible and therefore you can see that leadership can be exercised by different people in the same setting.

So, we are dealing with two different aspects in the context of leading amongst equals:

1 the function performed by leaders is clearly influenced by the task and the context in which it occurs
2 the range of leadership styles; individuals may operate in many different ways depending upon their own nature, values and beliefs and the characteristics of other members of the group. Some people will adopt a high profile and lead from the front assertively and yet others will lead more obscurely from the side, whilst others will exert an almost unrecognised influence from the back.

Using multiple leadership styles effectively is a complex and highly skilled role. It requires the meta leader and most people will not be able to do this. They will be more attuned to certain situations where like the 'one club golfer' their particular approach works. In complex peer based teams the skill is in recognising one of the demands of modern workforces – everyone can be a leader at different times and in different circumstances. Leadership is a dispersed, diffused capacity no longer resident in one individual. In leading amongst equals it is important to acknowledge that the sum of the collective leadership capacity is far greater than the restricted investment in a single individual and is required in modern settings.

Top tips

- In order to operate effectively as a leader amongst equals complex interactions need to be recognised and dealt with.
- Be clear about the demands of the task(s) or challenge(s) being taken on by the group.
- Understand the critical skills needed to tackle the task.
- Consider where these skills exist within team members.
- Recognise the contribution of the role and status of individual members of the team.
- Consider how far it is appropriate for the same person to act as a leader at all times.
- Consult with the group about roles required and the acceptability of someone taking a lead role in specific circumstances.
- Recognise the contribution of all to the team's success.
- Operate in a consultative and participative style so that peers feel they can make a contribution and are not inappropriately subordinate to another person.
- Set out a time period for a particular leadership role matched to the task or challenge, with a system for review of the identity of the leader.
- Be willing to contribute when in a follower role.
- Reflect whether the group is functioning effectively and if the leadership role is being fulfilled appropriately.

Frequently asked questions and answers

Q. *I have suggested several changes in my practice which we could all make that would improve our overall service to the patients. It has surprised me how much resistance this has met with from my partners and practice manager.*
A. It is likely that this is a well intentioned change but the leadership function you describe has failed to recognise the status and provision of your colleagues, expecting them to follow a set of recommendations. Your colleagues are likely to feel that as your equals with a similar stake in the service that your practice provides they should have been consulted before your proposals were made. Try a more open, consultative approach that draws people into recognising the problem(s) at an early stage in your action planning and commenting on, or proposing, some possible solutions which you could then include in your discussions.

Q. *We never seem to make progress as a team because people seem to be committed to their own ideas and are reluctant to support proposals made by others.*
A. It is likely that all members of your group feel that they have expertise and a legitimate contribution to make for solving any problem. Their expertise is likely

to be greater in certain areas than others. Therefore the process of leadership needs to acknowledge these differing qualities and ensure that when they are key the appropriate person has a lead role. This must be discussed and agreed in your team at the outset as a way of making sure that the leadership role is not seen as being dominant or antagonistic but allows everyone to play the leader role as and when it meets the needs of the situation.

Interactive exercise: finding an equally good way

Think about a group meeting when you have been present where individuals of similar status have come together to tackle a particular problem. Different ideas will have emerged as to how the issue should be dealt with.

Write down or think out what happened. Who led the group? How did they come to be recognised as the leader? How did their leadership role work out? Was it a smooth process or were there challenges or conflicts? Was the problem solved successfully? If so, how did the way that the leader performed add to the successful outcome(s)? If not, how did the way that the leader acted contribute to the unsuccessful outcome(s)? How could that leader have behaved differently to improve the effectiveness of the group, or resolution of the problem?

Now consider a group of equals to which you belong and a topic that you are wrestling with or are about to address. Work through the following possible ways of resolving the leadership issues:

• appoint a dominant leader and tell him or her to drive through a particular approach. How would this work? What is likely to happen?
• analyse the requirement of the task and seek to appoint sub-groups to discuss each issue and how they can be tackled. What might be helpful about such an approach and what might be the downside?
• discuss the skills and contributions that individuals feel they can make, and how to do it? Suggest you match the range of skills to the requirements of the task and ask key individuals to lead developments in their own area(s). What are the merits of this approach and why might leadership amongst equals be best fulfilled with this approach?

References

1   Plsek P, Greenhalgh T. The challenge of complexity in health care. *BMJ.* 2001; **323**: 625–8.
2   George J, Jones G. *Understanding and Managing Organisational Behaviour.* Reading Massachusetts: Addison-Wesley; 1999.
3   Williams S. *Evidence of the Contribution Leadership Development for Professional Groups Makes in Driving their Organisations Forward.* Berkhamsted: Henley Management Centre, Henley College; 2004.

Chapter 16

Growing new leaders

Robert Cragg

Introduction

The NHS has a long-standing history of identifying and nurturing people's leadership potential. In recent years the scale of leadership development has expanded to keep pace with the vast change in management programme currently being undertaken throughout the NHS. In spite of such positive intent on behalf of the NHS, 'effective' strategies for leadership development are scarce. There is no consensus model for how to do it.[1] The *'transformational'* model of leadership development however seems to be a good method to adopt, by defining the leadership skills that someone can acquire through training and reflection (*see* page 34).

This chapter provides insights for organisations that want to nurture or recruit new leaders, on how to identify, select and support those with the greatest leadership potential. This approach might suit a trust or a practice or other unit. It explores how organisations can help individuals to gain the mechanics of being a leader through learning and reflective practice to accelerate their acquisition of leadership skills.

> Live as if you were to die tomorrow. Learn as if you were to live forever.
> Mahatma Gandhi

How do we identify new leaders?

Identifying high quality leaders starts with good old-fashioned HR practice – designing a job description and person specification pertinent to the intended leadership role. Alongside it, you need a strong job outline that is tailored to your strategic plans and the organisation's recruitment framework. It should describe the potential leadership behaviours you envisage that indicate effective job performance.

Historically organisations have identified prospective leaders by subjectively assessing a person's personality and charisma at interview, a methodology strongly aligned to the trait theory model of leadership (*see* page 33).[2] Since the 1980s, recruitment practice has become more sophisticated, based on transformational and transactional leadership models (*see* page 34), with the specific approach adopted often reflecting the size of the recruiting organisation.

Competency based assessment centres are now virtually ubiquitous in the NHS, deployed to underpin leadership recruitment processes within NHS trusts. This format of recruitment is common for substantive roles, whereby the staffing complement enables individuals to make job applications for posts that are both external and internal to their organisation. In addition to traditional individual interviews, assessment centres of this kind typically use: in-tray exercises and group work simulating real life work-based scenarios, psychometric testing, and problem solving requiring numerical and written analyses. No assessment will ever capture a candidate's true character and competence, so the final decision still rests with the intuitive judgments of those on interview panels taking into account the assessment centre's findings.[2]

Smaller community teams and independent contractor practices may not have sufficient scope to recruit a new full-time leader, relying on internal part-time promotions or role extensions within the existing staff complement, to take on leadership responsibility. In such instances post holders are selected according to who volunteers or whose skills and competencies best match the intended job role(s). In such a close-knit environment assessment may be deemed unnecessary, as the practice or team leader is already aware of the candidate's potential. If a post is competitively contested then internal competency-based interviews and presentations are usually used in selection.

What should we look for in prospective leaders?

Organisations need to be conscious that leaders do not conform to any specific stereotype nor are they solely in the middle to late stages of their careers or necessarily already within the elite hierarchy. Instead you will find potential leaders across all age ranges and organisational ranks.[2] Naturally, no individual will have all the attributes of 'good leadership' (*see* Chapter 5), but potential new leaders will typically have such attributes as: creativity, high levels of motivation, emotional tact and a willingness to promote change.

Learning to lead

Learning and leadership development are inextricably linked. Kolb's learning cycle is a framework pertinent to the process of acquiring and fine-tuning leadership skills. When developing a new skill a leader needs to undergo a sequence of 'conceptualisation', 'experimentation', 'experience' and 'reflection' before they can master a new competency or behaviour.[3] Over time, the learning and knowledge assimilated with every cycle of successive experience will result in improved performance (*see* Figure 16.1).

Whilst the four stages naturally follow each other the start point is not fixed, but based on a person's previous knowledge and experience. The sequence may take hours or months to complete depending on the complexity of the task undertaken. Sometimes a single cycle may be required, whilst other times one sequence may be sufficient for someone to gain competence and confidence.

Effective learning requires a strong partnership between a person nurturing a new leader and the inexperienced leader themselves. Personal coaches need in-depth experience of the competency being developed. It is best if the type and content of the learning is matched to the inexperienced leader's learning style and specific needs. Honey and Mumford inspired by Kolb, likened each stage of

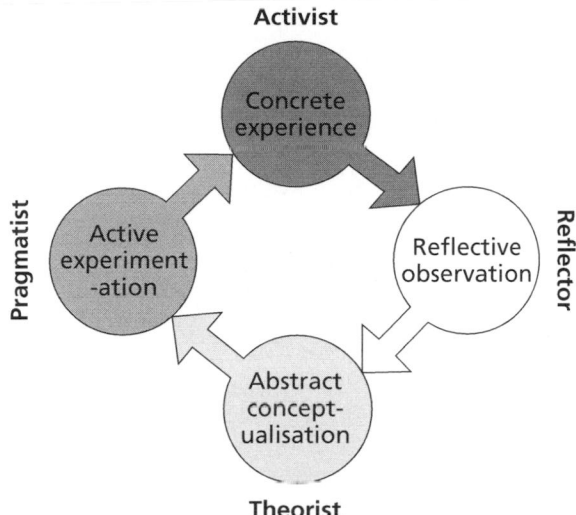

Figure 16.1 Kolb's Learning Cycle. Adapted from Kolb,[3] and Honey and Mumford.[4]

the learning sequence to a learning style: 'theorist' 'pragmatist' 'activist' and 'reflector'.[3,4] Whilst individuals have a specific preference for one or two of these learning styles, exposing them to all these formats is good practice.

A good leadership development programme will always be underpinned by a solid foundation in academic theory. New leaders need confidence to emerge from their peer group. Acquiring a detailed knowledge of their core business provides them with an edge so that they can start to exert a positive influence over their colleagues – and start to lead. Be it through a formal qualification or informal private reading or reflection, they need to assimilate a wide based knowledge of leadership theory, health policy and corporate functions.[5]

Experimenting with putting newfound knowledge into action is a key part of the learning cycle. Simulating real life leadership scenarios prior to enacting them pays dividends. The inexperienced leader will gain in confidence as they will have already practised a leadership role in situations likely to happen in real life and developed foresight as they anticipate how people will react and events unfold. Supported action learning sets are great ways to 'role play', in a safe and consequence free environment. The sort of tasks that are particularly pertinent to action learning of this kind are those requiring key leadership behaviours such as assertiveness, negotiation and influencing skills.

Whilst virtual simulations are helpful in honing strategies and visualising your approach, they are no substitute for real life experiences. New leaders require intensive exposure to wide scoping roles, to explore and identify the boundaries of their individual style. The wider the exposure, the steeper the learning curve, the more skills and perspectives they will obtain. Whilst those guiding their development as leaders should attempt to minimise risks from the novice leader learning to act in a leadership role, this should not be at the expense of them taking responsibility as leader – with the inevitable experiences of both success and failure.

Reflection is key

A key element of leadership development relies on the person's ability to develop and improve their skills and performance as a leader through the self-awareness that comes from reflection. There are many ways to facilitate reflective practice: personal reflection in private time, peer group learning sets, and from receiving personal coaching or mentoring.[6] The inexperienced leader will determine what works for them, often preferring one form of reflection to another. Leaders should not rely solely on internal reflection though, as the perspective provided by others such as colleagues, coaches and mentors can give them the insights they need about their leadership style and impact on others. Figure 16.2 captures a range of techniques that will aid reflection.

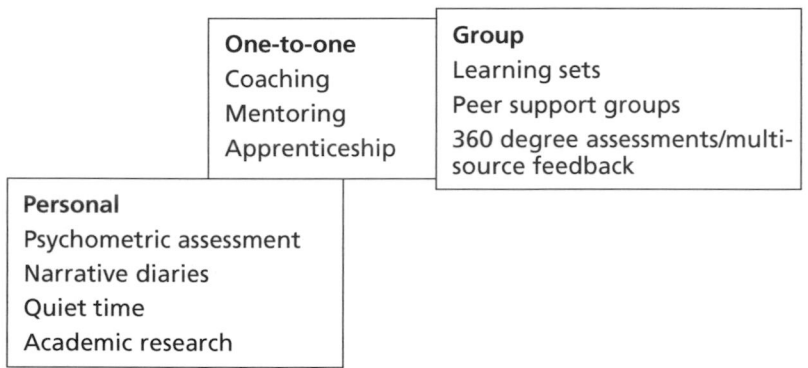

Figure 16.2 Vehicles for reflection.

The environment for leadership development

The design and delivery of leadership development programmes will vary according to different organisations' goals, the level of their investment and interest in the inexperienced leader, the new leader's prior experience and the priority that organisations give to developing and growing new leaders.[2] The infrastructure surrounding the inexperienced leader must provide intensive support and guidance if they are to take on significant responsibilities and rapidly grow into their leadership role. Those guiding their development should be of the right calibre with experience of training or supporting new leaders. Accreditation of the leadership development may be desirable, but is not essential.

Top tips

1 From the inexperienced leader's perspective:
  - as a prospective applicant for a senior leadership role you need to prepare for interviews and assessment centres by ensuring that you are aware of your relative strengths and weaknesses, and the extent to which you match the competency framework of the leader position
  - ensure that your *personal* and the *organisation's* developments are aligned.[2] Both streams of leadership development are essential to attain higher and

consistent levels of organisational performance as well as to develop your transferable leadership skills

- expose yourself to new learning experiences, taking on tasks outside your comfort zone in order to develop new competencies and experience new situations
- find a method of reflection that suits you so that reflecting on your performance as a leader becomes part of your daily working life. It would be good to find senior colleagues and/or peers with whom you feel comfortable reflecting and arrange to meet up.

2   From an NHS organisation's perspective:

- organisations should focus leadership roles upon specific outcomes. Leaders with unclear or non-challenging objectives can become de-motivated
- organisations need to learn from established leadership development programmes like the national 'NHS management training scheme', adapting them to suit local need
- those nurturing new leaders should harness the energy and fresh perspectives that potential leaders can bring
- a line manager who invests in the inexperienced leader will reap the rewards disproportionately, being able to share their workload and responsibility as the new leader grows within their role[2]
- whilst you should not expect new leaders to be running organisations from day one, they do need to have roles of real influence to aid their personal development and motivation
- organisations should focus on continuing professional development of those in pre-existing leadership roles, as well as provide leadership development for inexperienced leaders or new recruits. Too often there is inadequate support and training for people in established (clinical) leadership positions
- interim and post programme evaluations should assess the success of development activities and their delivery
- leadership development can provide a vehicle for cultural change. Leadership capacity needs to be proactively developed and new leaders encouraged; you cannot simply wait and expect leaders to emerge miraculously overnight.[2]

Frequently asked questions and answers

Q. *How do I raise my profile as a new leader?*
A. Networking is key. This could be both internal and external to your organisation. It will improve your career prospects and job effectiveness. Think of building working relations with your contemporaries and seniors across your trust or strategic health authority or in special interest groups or networks. Networking is often synonymous with a careerist approach, which does not sit comfortably with a more modest public sector ethos, so overcome your reservations and get on with it. Networking not only improves your visibility but also aids development by enhancing your knowledge of different systems and sectors.[5] Volunteering for tasks, and actively extending your areas of responsibility can also enhance your visibility to others in your organisation and beyond.

Q. *What are the benefits of having a coach or mentor and how do I obtain one?*
A. Both mentoring and coaching share the same basic premise. Both involve

supporting and guiding an individual through a learning and challenging process to help them to reach their full potential. Coaching is a great way to help someone develop insights into key leadership behaviours. Mentors take a more overarching approach to a person's personal development and career planning, exposing them to wider networks.[7,8] Coaches and mentors can offer more wide ranging sources of development compared to that within hierarchical organisational structures. This independence provides confidentiality and openness in the relationship between the person and their coach or mentor, which should be judgement free.[7] Whereas line managers are prescribed in relation to someone's employed post, coaches and mentors can specifically fit with the learning style and needs of the inexperienced leader. Best if you select your mentor or coach on the basis of those whom you respect or see as a role model. It can be intimidating for you to ask senior members of your organisation if they could assume a mentoring or coaching role for you, but they are often flattered to be approached – so go ahead and ask them.

Interactive exercise: learning to cycle

Turn back to Figure 16.1 and look at Kolb's learning cycle upon which this exercise is based.

- Agree a learning need relating to a specific competency associated with leadership, with someone who is encouraging you to grow as a new leader – this could be your leadership development programme lead, a continuing professional development tutor, an interested colleague or your line manager. The competency identified will be either linked to a new area of work for you or a current area of work in which you require additional development.
- Now study the theory behind the chosen competency. This will involve self-directed learning – for instance, academic reading, shadowing an established leader, or observing colleagues who already have that demonstrable competence.
- Once you have acquired the relevant theoretical knowledge you need to prepare for the real experience through active experimentation. Talk through your strategy with your adviser or guide, visualise your use of the new competency in the context of the specific task and stakeholders involved. Explore all possible scenarios and outcomes.
- Now you need the autonomy and time to enact your strategy through your concrete experience. Rope in your adviser or guide in supporting you through real life experiences, assisting in problem solving, providing you with challenge, feedback and advice.
- When you reflect afterwards think of both positive and negative aspects of your performance and how others responded and events unfolded. Use your reflection to identify gaps in your performance and plan how to remedy any weaknesses in future. Store how you did as a benchmark for comparing with your experiences in the future.
- Once you and your adviser are happy that you have indeed obtained the competency, reflect on this learning experience together and evaluate its benefit as a framework to guide your continuing learning plan and related activities.

References

1   Alimo-Metcalfe B, Lawler J. Leadership development in UK companies at the beginning of the twenty-first century: lessons for the NHS? *J Manag Med*. 2001; **15** (4–5): 387–404.

2   Adair J. *Effective Leadership*. 2nd ed. London: Pan Books Ltd; 1988.

3   Kolb D. *Experiential Learning: experience as the source of learning and development*. New Jersey: Prentice-Hall; 1984.

4   Honey P, Mumford A. *Manual of Learning Styles*. London: Peter Honey; 1982.

5   Hardacre J. *Leadership at every level: a practical guide for managers*. London: Health Service Journal Management Academy; 2001.

6   Boud D, Keogh R, Walker D. *Reflection: turning experience into learning*. London: Kogan Page; 1996.

7   Parsloe E. *The Manager as Coach and Mentor*. 2nd ed. Management shapers series. London: CIPD Publications; 2001.

8   Megginson D, Clutterbuck D, Garvey B, *et al. Mentoring in Action: a practical guide for managers*. 2nd ed. London: Kogan Page; 2005.

Index

Adair, J 35
adverse incidents 17–18
  and poor performance 78–9
  use of 'decision trees' 79–80
  see also mistakes and errors
Alban-Metcalfe, J 34
Alimo-Metcalfe, B 33, 34
Allman, S 98
appraisals 43
  introducing to staff 72
  undertaking 70–2
approaches and concepts of leadership 1–3
assertiveness 25–6
  key tips 28
assumptions 10–11
attributes and descriptors of leadership
    16–17

Bass, BM 34
behavioural approaches 2–3
Belbin, RM 49–50
blame cultures 77–8
body language, and assertiveness 28
British Association of Medical Managers,
    'Fit to Lead' programme 21
'broken record' techniques 28–9

challenging and motivating skills 9
change management 55–61, 85–9
  key tips 87–8
  change adoption rates 56–9
  communication skills 86–7
  emotional and behavioural challenges
      85–7
  encouraging involvement 12, 44
  implementation models 56–8
  interactive exercises 60–1, 88–9
  key tasks 55–6
  morale and motivation issues 87–8
  overcoming barriers 55, 60
  sustaining developments 56
  team resistance 11, 60, 88
  see also organisational change
characteristics of leadership 2
charismatic leadership 101–2
Churchill, Winston 34
coaching 106, 108, 109–10
communication skills 7–12
  key tips 11

challenging and motivating abilities 9
conflict management 9
creating rapport 9
during change 86–7
interpreting meanings 10–11
negotiation and influencing others 9–10
competency–based approaches 2, 34–8,
    105–6
  key tips 36–7
  frameworks and models 35–6
  and performance 37
  theoretical background 33–5
complaints management
  anonymous accusations 74
  grievance handling 72, 74
confidence issues 4
confidentiality, in significant event analysis
    18
conflict management 9
context and conditions of leadership 3, 42,
    102–3
control issues 27, 30, 86
  coping with outside demands 30, 86
  paperwork management 26
  see also time management
Covey, SR 97
cultural familiarity 10
cultural 'norms' 49
culture of openness 77–8
'cycle of change' model (Procheska *et al.*)
    57–9

decision-making skills 26
  interactive exercises 30–1
  key tips 27–8
  tools and techniques 79–80
delegation 65
deletions 10–11
developmental approaches 41–2
'Diffusion of innovation' model (Rogers)
    56–7
distortions 11
Dye, CF and Garman, AN 35–6

effectiveness
  key tips 27–8
  and team work 47–52
  tools and techniques 25–31
environmental considerations 42

equal opportunities 42
  dealing with grievances 74
errors *see* mistakes and errors
'exceptional leadership' framework (Dye
  and Garman) 35–6
expertise development 21–2

feedback, and learning needs 15, 16,
  18–20
feelings and emotions 9
'Fit to Lead' programme (BAMM) 21
'forming/storming/norming/performing'
  phases 48–9, 87
frameworks for leadership 35–6
  see also NHS Leadership Qualities
    Framework (LQF)
funding training 45

Gandhi, Mahatma 105
generalisations 11
Goodwin, Neil 25, 42, 91
Government initiatives, managing
  demands 30
grievances 72, 74
group development processes 48–9
  see also teams
'group-think' 49

Hay Group, *In Tune with the Team* study
  (2006) 2–3
health needs 27
health problems, and performance 81
Honey, P and Mumford, A 106–7

ideas and proposals
  methods of introducing 10, 12
  see also change management
identifying leaders 105–6
In Tune with the Team study (Hay Group
  2006) 2–3
incident analysis 17–18
  'decision tree' 79–80
  and poor performance 78–80
  see also mistakes and errors
influencing others 9–10
innovators 56
interactive exercises
  assessing decision–making skills 30–1
  change management 60–1, 88–9
  competencies analysis 37–8
  identifying learning needs 22
  Kolb's learning cycle 110
  on management/leadership roles 100
  peer meetings 104

performance concerns 82
problem resolution skills 82
research leadership 95
stressful events 75
team development 12
time management 67
under-performance management 45
interruptions 65

job satisfaction 71
Johnson, S 55

Kolb's learning cycle 106–7, 110
Kouzes, J and Poisner, B 7

language use
  creating rapport 9
  deletions, generalisations and distortions
    10–11
leadership
  attributes and descriptors 16–17
  cf. 'management' 2, 97–100
  communication skills 7–12
  concepts and approaches 1–3, 33–8
  frameworks 2, 21, 35–6
  general tips 3
  identification and recognition 105–10
  learning needs 15–22
  motives for undertaking 26
  peer relations 101–4
  qualities 1–2, 4, 7
  staff development and management
    41–3
  team working 47–52
  theories and models 33–8
Leadership Qualities Framework (LQF) 2,
  21, 35
'learned helplessness' 58
learning cultures 71
learning cycle (Kolb) 106–7, 110
learning needs 15–22, 106–10
  key tips 20–1, 108–9
  environmental considerations 108
  identifying needs 15–16
  identifying potential 105–6
  lack of recognition 17
  time constraints 21
  use of mistake evaluations 17
  use of multisource feedback 18–20, 108
  use of reflection 108
  use of self-assessment 16–17
  use of significant event audit 17–18
  see also staff training
learning styles 106–7

learning to lead 106–10
  organisation perspectives 109

Machin, J 51
management, cf. leadership 2, 97–100
'Management Team Wheel' (Margerison
    and McCann) 50
Margerison, CJ and McCann, DJ 50
meanings, interpretation skills 10–11
medical errors *see* mistakes and errors
meetings
  chairing skills 69–70
  interpreting meanings 10–11
  language use 10–11
  peer interactions 101–4
  and team work 48
  time management 66–7
mentoring 108, 109–10
mistakes and errors
  blame cultures 77–8
  costs and impacts 77
  identifying incidents 78–9
  learning opportunities 17
misunderstandings 10–11
models and theories of leadership 33–4
motivation
  during change 87–8
  influencing others 9, 11–12, 87–8
  self assessments 26
  and staff performance 70–1
multidisciplinary teams 47, 49
  see also teams
multisource feedback 18–20

National Patient Safety Agency 79–80
negotiation skills 9–10
networking 109
neurolinguistic programming 10–11
NHS changes
  coping strategies 44
  managing demands 30
NHS Leadership Qualities Framework
    (LQF) 2, 21, 35
'novice to expert' learning pathway 21–2

organisational change
  coping strategies 44
  emotional and behavioural responses 85–7
  managing demands 30
  see also change management
organisational management 42–3
organisational skills 69–75
  key tips 72–4
  chairing meetings 69–70

dealing with grievances 72, 74
  undertaking appraisals 70–2
outcomes-based approaches 2–3

paperwork, control measures 26
peer group learning sets 108
peer meetings 101–4
performance concerns 43
  diagnosing causes 79–80
  health problems 81
  identifying problems 78–9
  information sources 81
  interactive exercises 82
  management tips 43–4, 80–1
  rehabilitation and support 81–2
  see also appraisals
personal effectiveness
  key tips 27–8
  tools and techniques 25–31
personal fitness 27
personal qualities 1–2, 4, 7
personality types
  and change 56–7
  and stress 27
  and team roles 50
Plsek, P and Greenhalgh, T 101
policy directives, on team working 47
poor management 43–4
poor performance *see* performance
    concerns
problem analysis 80
  see also incident analysis; performance
    concerns
problem resolution 77–82
  key tips 80–1
  cultural considerations 77–8
  diagnosing cause 79–80
  identifying poor performance 78–9
  incident reporting barriers 78
  interactive exercises 82
processes 42, 48
proposals and ideas, methods of
    introducing 10, 12

Ramsden, P 16–17
rapport with others 9
reflection 108
research leadership 91–5
  key tips 93–4
  competencies and tasks 91–3
  interactive exercises 95
  patenting and copyright issues 94
  peer collaborations 94
  resource management 92

reward systems 60
Rogers, EM 56–7
role modelling 36
role play 107
roles, within teams 49–50
Roosevelt, Theodore 69
'root cause analysis' 79–80

saying 'NO' 28
self-assessment, learning needs 16–17
sex discrimination, dealing with grievances
    74
significant event analysis (SEA) 17–18
    see also incident analysis
situational leadership 33–4
staff development 41–3
staff mix 42
staff training 42–3
    funding 45
'storming/reforming/norming/performing'
    48–9, 87
strengths and weaknesses analysis 16–17, 37
stress
    management concerns 26–7, 30
    and performance 81
stressful events 75, 81

task, defined 48
task management 26
'task—team—individual' leadership
    framework (Adair) 35
task-related processes 48
Taylor, Ros 1
team 'players' 51
teams 47–52
    change resistance 11
    cultural 'norms' 49
    decision-making 49
    definitions 47–8

development 12, 48–9, 51–2
    interactive exercises 12, 51–2
    key processes 48
    lack of involvement 12
    leadership tips 50–1
    maintenance issues 48–9
    management tips 50–1
    roles 51–2
    uses 51
theories and models of leadership 33–4
360 degree feedback 18–20
time management 63–7
    interactive exercises 67
    key tips 66
    and learning needs 21
    prioritising tasks 63–5
    and work flow 26
Tolstoy, Leo 85
training
    funding 45
    leadership needs 15–22
    staff needs 42–3
trait theory 33, 35, 101–2
transactional leadership 34, 35
transformational leadership 33, 34, 35,
    105
transtheoretical model of change
    (Procheska et al.) 57–9
triangulation assessments 15–16
'21st Century' leadership framework
    (Alimo–Metcalfe) 35

under-performance 43
    interactive exercises 45
    management tips 43–4

virtual simulations 107

work flow management 26